Advancing Nursing Practice in Pain Management

Advancing Nursing Practice in Pain Management

Edited by

ELOISE CARR
Associate Dean Postgraduate Students
School of Health & Social Care
Bournemouth University

MANDY LAYZELL
Lecturer Practitioner
Advanced Specialist Nurse
Acute Pain Team
Poole Hospital NHS Foundation Trust

MARTIN CHRISTENSEN
Senior Lecturer
School of Health & Social Care
Bournemouth University

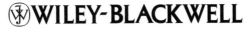

A John Wiley & Sons, Ltd., Publication

This edition first published 2010
© Blackwell Publishing Ltd

Blackwell Publishing was acquired by John Wiley & Sons in February 2007. Blackwell's publishing programme has been merged with Wiley's global Scientific, Technical, and Medical business to form Wiley-Blackwell.

Registered office
John Wiley & Sons Ltd, The Atrium, Southern Gate, Chichester, West Sussex, PO19 8SQ, United Kingdom

Editorial office
9600 Garsington Road, Oxford, OX4 2DQ, United Kingdom
2121 State Avenue, Ames, Iowa 50014-8300, USA

For details of our global editorial offices, for customer services and for information about how to apply for permission to reuse the copyright material in this book please see our website at www.wiley.com/wiley-blackwell.

Library of Congress Cataloging-in-Publication Data

Advancing nursing practice in pain management / edited by Eloise Carr, Martin Christensen, Mandy Layzell.
    p. ; cm.
Includes bibliographical references and index.
ISBN 978-1-4051-7699-6 (pbk. : alk. paper)
1. Pain–Nursing.   2. Nursing.   I. Carr, Eloise C. J.   II. Christensen, Martin.   III. Layzell, Mandy.
    [DNLM: 1. Pain–nursing. WY 160.5 A2445 2010]
RT87.P35.A38 2010
610.73–dc22

                                                                          2009030832

A catalogue record for this book is available from the British Library.

Set in 10/12.5pt Times New Roman by Aptara® Inc., New Delhi, India
Printed and bound in Malaysia by KHL Printing Co Sdn Bhd

1   2010

Contents

Contributors' biographies

Name Christine M. Barnes
Affiliation Nurse Practioners for Pain Management Services, Chesterfield Royal Hospital NHS Foundation Trust
Short biography Christine M. Barnes is a nurse practitioner in pain services at Chesterfield Royal Hospital. She has been working in pain services for 7 years. She is herself an acupuncturist, a nurse prescriber and has supervised and mentored many nurses towards competency in acupuncture.

Name Elaine Beddingham
Affiliation Clinical Placement Learning Facilitator (formally Pain Nurse Practitioner), Education Centre, Chesterfield Royal Hospital NHS Foundation Trust
Short biography Elaine Beddingham is now a clinical placement learning facilitator and formally a nurse practitioner in pain management for 11 years. She is an experienced acupuncturist and has been involved in the development and delivery of acupuncture courses. She is also a teacher and a mentor to nurses learning to practise acupuncture.

Name Paul Bibby
Affiliation Operations Director, Pain Management Solutions; Honorary Lecturer, The University of Cardiff; Honorary Research Fellow, Sheffield Hallam University
Short biography Paul has worked in pain management services for 15 years. Having set up the acute pain service in Doncaster, he went on to develop the role of consultant pain nurse at Sherwood Forest Hospital NHS Foundation Trust. During this time he began to focus on the development of community-based pain services which led him to form Pain Management Solutions Ltd which now provides pain clinics in primary care for a number of PCTs in South Yorkshire and Nottinghamshire.

Name Dr. Dee Burrows
Affiliation Consultant Nurse & Managing Director, PainConsultants Limited
Short biography Dee is a consultant nurse, founder and director of PainConsultants Limited and also contributes to the Buckinghamshire PCT Chronic Pain and Fatigue Management Services. She works predominantly with people with chronic pain delivering pain management and pain education programmes and also has an interest in the impact of pain upon families.

Name: Eloise Carr
Affiliation: Associate Dean Postgraduate Students, School of Health & Social Care, Bournemouth University
Short biography Eloise has a clinical background in surgical nursing and is passionate about how education and research can be used to improve patient care. Recent research includes GP's management of low back pain, anxiety before surgery, imaging and back pain, and pain and day case surgery. She has published many articles and book chapters, developed pain open learning material, several textbooks and a video. She serves on Council for the British Pain Society and chairs a Special Interest Group in pain education.

Name Martin Christensen
Affiliation Senior Lecturer, Bournemouth House, Bournemouth University
Short biography Martin Christensen is a senior lecturer at Bournemouth University. He has 20 years of experience in critical care nursing and divides his time between teaching and supporting critical care nursing practice as a member of the clinical education team at Southampton General Hospital. His PhD centred around the advancement of nursing practice in critical care from which he was able to develop a knowledge integration model using aspects of reflection, work-based learning and clinical supervision. His current interests are advancing and advanced nursing practice and the assessment of clinical practice using the novice to expert model of skill acquisition.

Name Gillian Chumbley
Affiliation Consultant Nurse, Pain Service, Imperial College Healthcare NHS Trust
Short biography Gillian Chumbley is the consultant nurse for the pain service at Imperial College Healthcare NHS Trust and leads a team of nurses who manage both acute and chronic pain. She has 15 years of experience working in pain management and completed her PhD, evaluating the patient's experience of patient-controlled analgesia, at St George's Hospital Medical School in 2001. Her recent interest has been in the use of low-dose ketamine for uncontrolled post-operative pain.

Name: Felicia Cox
Affiliation Senior Nurse, Pain Management, Royal Brompton & Harefield NHS Trust
Short biography Felicia is responsible for the management of nurse-led acute and chronic pain services in the trust, and also acts as the lead clinician for the service as a whole, directing resources and raising the service profile through publication, audit and research.

Name Ruth Day
Affiliation PhD Student, Bournemouth University; Consultant Nurse, PainConsultants Limited
Short biography Ruth has worked in the area of pain management for over 14 years. She has established acute pain and chronic pain services and is currently researching in the area of back pain.

Name Christine M. Haigh
Affiliation Nurse Practioners for Pain Management Services, Chesterfield Royal Hospital NHS Foundation Trust
Short biography Christine M. Haigh is a nurse practitioner in pain services at Chesterfield Royal Hospital. She has been working in pain services for 6 years. She is an experienced acupuncturist. Her particular area of interest is clinical governance and how this impacts on day-to-day running of an acupuncture service.

Name Ruth H. Heafield
Affiliation Nurse Consultant and Manager, Pain Management Services, Chesterfield Royal Hospital NHS Foundation Trust
Short biography Ruth has been working in pain management since 1994. She cares for those with both acute and chronic pain and her constant challenge is to develop services, in the current financial climate, using the strength of both traditional and complementary therapies together. Specific interests include those with acute on chronic pain and substance misusers. She is involved in national pain management groups, including the development of the essence of care benchmarks for pain management.

Name Mandy Layzell
Affiliation Advanced Specialist Nurse, Acute Pain Team, Poole Hospital NHS Foundation Trust
Short biography Mandy has been working in acute pain management since 1998, and in addition, over the last 8 years her role has been split between clinical practice and education. Her current role involves leading a team of nurses caring for hospital-based patients with both acute and chronic pain needs. Her areas of interests lie in education for health professionals and patients, and non-pharmacological strategies for managing pain.

Name Eileen Mann
Affiliation Recently retired Lecturer in Pain Management at School of Health & Social Care, Bournemouth University, and Nurse Consultant in Pain Management at Poole Hospital NHS Trust
Short biography Eileen's career in pain management spanned the UK and Australia. She was a vanguard of change and improvement in pain and provided a role model for others. She held a lecturer–practitioner role at Bournemouth University and was jointly responsible for developing innovative e-learning around pain management. Although recently retired Eileen retains an interest in pain, currently writing and reviewing journal articles.

Name Ann Taylor
Affiliation Napp Sponsored Senior Lecturer in Pain Research and Education Department of Anaesthetics, Cardiff University
Short biography Ann is a senior lecturer within the department and currently a director for three MSc courses – pain, advanced surgical practice and critical care. She has authored the commissioning directives for chronic pain for Wales and now

chairs the advisory board which is helping and supporting local health boards in implementing these directives. She is currently undertaking her PhD looking at fear and anxiety in relation to pain management programmes using fMRI. She is involved in a number of educational initiatives around supporting clinicians in their roles as educationalists.

Name Trudy Towell
Affiliation Consultant Nurse Pain Management, The Midlands NHS Treatment Centre, Burton upon Trent
Short biography Trudy's career in pain management has spanned nearly 30 years. She has been instrumental in developing the UK 'Pain Network' for nurses working in pain management. Her clinical career focused on the development of pain services, and more recently she has led the development of nurse prescribing and setting up acupuncture clinics. She has recently retired from consultant nurse in pain management/anaesthesia, Nottingham University Hospitals NHS Trust and Queen's Medical Centre Campus. She has consistently contributed to education and research.

Foreword 1

Advancing Nursing Practice in Pain Management is an innovative reference text that profiles nursing leadership in improving pain management practices in the UK. The editors themselves are well-known leaders in advancing the pain agenda. They clarify in Chapter 1 the nature of advanced practice as the integration of knowing-how-why-what and knowing-that with the advanced nurse practitioner as the practical exemplar of this transition. Outstanding models are provided for nurses who have been entrepreneurs in advancing pain practices and who reflect on the successes and challenges of their journey.

This book provides outstanding examples of successful initiatives lead by nurses that resulted in changes in acute and persistent pain management practices in diverse contexts, from procedures to programmes. Innovations focusing on pharmacological interventions and the health professionals involved can be very challenging and excellent strategies are outlined in Chapters 2, 3, 5 and 10. As well, the chapters on nurse-led clinics/programmes developed to meet the needs of people who have insufficient access or assistance to manage their pain problem are very helpful. Several authors provide readers with samples of tools and strategies they have developed to facilitate their programmes (Chapters 4, 5, 8, 9, 10 and 11). The transparency of the shared reflections involved in the project preparation, development and implementation in each chapter is refreshing and provides a realistic guide for those wishing to do something similar.

The editors have successfully captured the nursing contribution to advancing practice in pain management using a diversity of initiatives as exemplars. The stories differ, but common themes are evident throughout. Layzell emphasises that change requires motivation and a commitment to work differently (Chapter 2). Chumbley suggests that both a working knowledge of scientific evidence and good interprofessional relationships are essential for new directions, along with audit data to provide evidence of benefit (Chapter 3). Cox also underlines the importance of involving multidisciplinary teams whose members may share interests but who bring diverse knowledge, skills and experience (Chapter 5). Several authors emphasise that involving multidisciplinary colleagues is fundamental to the development and success of any project. To address the need for team involvement and a common understanding of roles, Taylor outlines an interprofessional pain course that can be accessed on-line (Chapter 11).

This book is unique in presenting pragmatic approaches that have resulted in successful nurse-led pain management initiatives. The editors emphasise that advancing practice is a developmental process and their encouragement of authors to be honest about the highs and lows of the process is admirable. The resulting chapters offer insight into important and innovative nurse-led pain management initiatives that will be models for the readers. I highly recommend this book as a resource to anyone wishing to be innovative and entrepreneurial in changing pain management practices.

Judy Watt-Watson RN PHD
University of Toronto, Canada

Foreword 2

Advancing Nursing Practice in Pain Management provides an important resource for all nurses seeking to develop their practice and move towards the pinnacle of the clinical career pathway in nursing. This book provides a wealth of insights and practice expertise with regard to caring for people in pain that will be of value to the individual generalist and specialist practitioner, the nurse working within the context of the inter-disciplinary team, and across a range of different patient pathways where pain management is a cross-cutting theme. More generally, it provides interesting and valuable learning for nurses working with innovation and who are interested in the processes of entrepreneurship because of the models it describes for introducing and sustaining entrepreneurial practice in pain services.

The book illustrates a continuum of examples of nurses challenging boundaries and barriers. These range from pushing the boundaries of everyday nursing practice in acute hospital and primary health settings; maintaining patient safety; developing nurse-led clinics and whole programmes of pain management; through ensuring that organisational and service systems sustain quality care across organisational boundaries within and across hospital, community, private and public sectors.

The management of pain is one of the most central and essential aspects of nursing practice. Although the primary aim is about relieving suffering, this aim is also a prerequisite for achieving a range of other positive health and social outcomes. Skilled pain management has great potential for enabling patients to feel positively different but also enables them, as a consequence, to get on with their everyday activities. This in turn impacts on how they experience the quality of their life. The consequence of not getting this right results in a burden not just for the individual and those important to them, but also for the society.

Pain management has come a long way in the last two decades and nursing has been at the fore of many of these developments. The contributors to this book are drawn from this ilk.

It is good to see that developments in pain management are not just translated into practice but also into education curricula – as it is through education programmes that best practice can be promoted and sustained. Whilst there is always a need for systematic, rigorous and continuous evaluation of nursing practice, where innovation and development are concerned, then this need is particularly important if innovations and practical strategies that work are to be disseminated quickly. Many of the chapters therefore focus on evaluation and audit. Expertise in evaluation is essential if measurable difference to the patient's experience of pain and related outcomes are to be established. Innovation needs to be judged in relation to not just evidence-based standards and competences but also key criteria and indicators linked to the standards that patients and users can expect.

The ability to evaluate innovations in practice and to implement findings in an ongoing way is the hallmark of nurses who are operating at the top of their clinical career ladder. Such nurses have expertise not just in providing person-centred, safe and effective care but also in developing systems that sustain this. The focus on nurse entrepreneurship in the book enables the reader to benefit from expertise in this area – a number of tools such as business cases and evaluation strategies are provided to this end. Regardless of whether readers wish to establish businesses themselves, the expertise shared in this area will help readers understand the business context in which we work and the arguments that will need to be made for nurse-led initiatives in any setting.

The framework applied to the content of the book is advancing nursing practice. The editors state a deliberate focus on knowledge translation and knowledge use in practice rather than knowledge generation – an excellent aim as this area continues to be one of the main challenges to effective nursing practice. The book's emphasis on 'know-how' that builds on 'know-that' and integrates this into practice can be described in another way as blending the different types of knowledge necessary to guide practical action in the workplace. It includes working with evidence from research, evidence from knowing the patient and knowing the situation in which care takes place, with knowledge from systematically reflecting on one's own experience, expertise and actions within the workplace. These actions need to be constantly exposed to critique and inquiry through peer review as this is at the heart of effective practice in nursing. When this skill set is developed to the highest level then nursing is most sophisticated in the articulation of its contribution, most accountable for its actions and most able to articulate the nuances of expertise from which others can learn.

Some of the chapters have endeavoured to use vignettes around the patient's experience combined with an analysis of nursing interventions and outcomes to begin to demonstrate the potential for this approach. Authors generally have endeavoured to reflect on these advancements for the benefit of those reading the book who would wish to glean every aspect of the contributors' expertise as well as the lessons learnt when introducing innovations around pain management.

The driving force underpinning all chapters is experienced by the reader as a dedicated and committed zest for finding solutions and improvements in pain management for patients wherever they are. I have no doubt that this book will influence nurses working within the area of pain management and will help them to learn from the valuable experience of the authors and their stories. These stories describe how the authors have advanced nursing practice, dismantled the barriers that practitioners face on a daily basis and achieved genuine improvement in the patient's experience.

Kim Manley PHD; MN; BA; RN; DIP N(LOND); RGNT; PGCEA; CBE
Head of Practice Development, Royal
College of Nursing

Preface

This book has been written over a period of time where health and social care is continuing to change, experiencing a continuing squeeze on resources and adapting to a burgeoning and complex demand on its services. Over the past few years, UK Health policy has been encouraging nurses to take a lead role in the development and provision of services. A recent commission on the 'Future of Nursing and Midwifery' has been launched with an explicit aim of providing information to maximise opportunities for nurses to control services and policy direction. At the time of going to print, the eagerly anticipated competencies from the Nursing and Midwifery Council have yet to be published. The RCN guide to the Advanced Nurse Practitioners (2008) had already provided domains and competencies and the Prime Minister's Commission of the future of nursing and midwifery which explicitly aimed to help put nurses in control of services had just been launched. For the focus on pain management the timely publication of the Chief Medical Officer's Report, which includes a compelling chapter on the prevalence of chronic pain and recommendations for action (DH 2009), could not have been better. Many of the issues appear in several chapters where the focus highlights a lack of service provision for those with chronic pain and reveals a real commitment to filling the gap to meet the needs of this neglected group.

One of the aims of this book has been to showcase the development and evaluation of innovative examples of pain management initiatives which have been led by nurses. Quite often they will have shared these developments through their presentations at local, national and sometimes international conferences. However, these presentations rarely have time to give real insight into how they developed the service, their challenges and how they overcame them. This book aims to provide a more considered platform as well as synthesise their advanced practice contributions across the different arenas in which they work.

We anticipate that this book will be a timely addition to the discussions regarding the nature of advancing nursing practice and, in particular, to those involved in the management of pain. We believe that it is a rich and inspirational collection from nurses who have taken forward the development of services and transparently shared their journey.

Eloise Carr

References

Advanced Nurse Practitioners, 2008. *An RCN Guide to the Advanced Nurse Practitioner Role, Competencies and Programme Accreditation*. London: Royal College of Nursing.

Department of Health, 2009. *On the State of Public Health – The Chief Medical Officer's Annual Report*. London: DH.

Acknowledgements

We would like to take the opportunity to thank Clive Andrewes who provided a huge support in the early discussions and development of this book. His commitment and encouragement for the concepts embedded in the heart of this book shaped its course.

Chapter 1
Introduction to advancing practice in pain management

Eloise Carr and Martin Christensen

Introduction

Textbooks concerned with 'advanced practice' for nursing are frequently preoccupied with discussions of theory. It is a popular subject as a quick internet search on 'advanced practice' or 'advanced nursing' reveals a plethora of books: at least 140, with many focusing on discrete areas of practice, e.g. older people, gastroenterology, surgery and oncology. Beyond those with a clinical focus there are books which only consider the legal aspects, research or evaluation. For this book we are solely interested in the 'translation' of advanced knowledge and skills for practice. The gap between theory and practice, in our opinion, has been exacerbated by the lack of published work telling the stories by those who do this innovative and ground-breaking work. In this book we bring these innovators to tell their story of the development, running and evaluation of a service, which has advanced our understanding and care of people in pain.

Before moving to these important contributions, we need to briefly review our position and understanding of what constitutes 'advanced' or indeed 'advancing practice' as well as cover a brief historical review of growth in the UK and globally. It is also important to offer definitions and differentiate between these roles and others such as the clinical nurse specialist and nurse practitioner.

The book explicitly sets the context of advancing practice in pain management, and therefore it is important to define pain and give an overview of the prevalence of pain in acute and community settings. This raises a number of issues relating to the challenges or barriers affecting the potential to deliver excellent pain management. Many of these difficulties appear in the chapters but often offer solutions.

Advanced practice

In the UK the profound changes in the National Health Service (NHS) coupled with changes in the scope of professional practice are making it possible for nurses to challenge professional boundaries and create and adopt new roles and responsibilities throughout the health care sector (Wilson-Barnett *et al.* 2000; McGee & Castledine

2003). Central to these changes has been the continual development of the advanced nurse practitioner.

The concept of advancing practice is central to the development of nursing practice and has been seen to take on many different forms depending on its use in context. To many it has become synonymous with the work of the advanced or expert practitioner; others have viewed it as a process of continuing professional development and skills acquisition (Wilson-Barnett *et al.* 2000; Por 2008). Moreover, it is becoming closely linked with practice development (Jenkins & White 2001; Jackson *et al.* 2003). This is where the concept of advancing nursing practice may be ambiguous and confusing, and some of the ambiguity perhaps derives from the inability to effectively define advancing and advanced practice.

It is difficult to discuss advanced practice without reference to the advanced practitioner because the concept and the individual are inextricably linked by the common theme of advanced knowledge and skills. In defining the advanced practitioner and giving an indication of the underlying foundation of advanced practice, the International Council of Nurses (2006, p. 12) suggested that the advanced practitioner is:

> ...a registered nurse who has acquired the expert knowledge base, complex decision making skills and clinical competencies for expanded practice.

In an earlier mission statement, the United Kingdom Central Council (1996) intimated that advanced practitioners have an eclectic knowledge base, are grounded in practice and support education and research. McGee and Castledine (2003) have further suggested that advanced nursing practice is a state of professional maturity, one in which practitioners are pioneering innovators and developers of health care. Others give differing accounts of advanced practice and the advanced practitioner, but, in essence, the qualities that are inherent within this role revolve around developing professional leadership, higher levels of scholarly enquiry, research, consultation, higher levels of autonomous practice, interprofessional team working and an acknowledgement of the wider political agenda (Dunn 1997; Fulbrook 1998; Woods 1999; Atkins & Ersser 2000; Davis & Hughes 2002; Royal College of Nursing 2003; Thompson & Watson 2003; Castledine 2004; Por 2008).

Where the advanced practitioner role is defined more in line with the personal attributes and abilities of individuals in providing expert care, the essence of advanced practice appears to centre on the continual ongoing acquisition of 'new' knowledge and skills to enhance and complement previous theoretical and practical knowing. This suggests that advanced practice is part of a continuum of advanced and advancing development (Jamieson *et al.* 2002; Scholes 2006). However, the problem with the nature of knowledge that defines advanced practice is that it either is heavily focused on a scientific research base or is deeply embedded in practice (Rolfe 1998); ideally it should encompass and enhance both. Rolfe (1998) constructed a typology of nursing knowledge (Table 1.1) that incorporates scientific, experiential and personal domains, and further characterised these into either theoretical (knowing-that) or practical knowledge (knowing-how). Schon (1983) called this 'knowing-in-action', which is steeped in the practical knowing of the here and now.

Table 1.1   Typology of advanced nursing practice (Rolfe 1998, p. 221)

Knowledge domain	Theoretical knowledge (knowing-that)	Practical knowledge (knowing-how)
Scientific knowledge	Things that are known: discovered from books, journals or lectures	Things that can be done: learnt from books, journals, guidelines or protocols of care
Experiential knowledge	Things that are known: discovered through own experience	Things that can be done: based on experience
Personal knowledge	Things that are known: which relate to specific situations or particular people, discovered through own experience	Things that can be done: which relate to specific situations or particular people

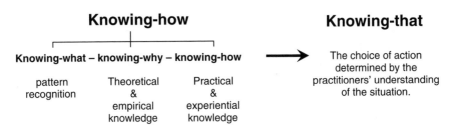

Figure 1.1   An alternative knowing-how and knowing-that knowledge framework.

These may not reflect the overlapping nature of advanced practice and we suggest that knowing-how knowledge consists of three distinct variables that portray the knowledge inherent in advancing and advanced practice and contain both content and process knowledge (Christensen 2009). These include knowing-how, which incorporates the practical and experiential knowledge; knowing-why, the theoretical and empirical knowledge; and knowing-what, which is pattern recognition knowledge reminiscent of Benner's (1984) expert model. If these were reproduced into a framework of knowledge acquisition, knowing-that could actually be the action undertaken by the practitioner based on a full and comprehensive understanding of the situation (Figure 1.1), which can only be achieved through a culmination of knowing-how, -what and -why.

One area of particular interest is the knowing-what (pattern recognition) element of knowing-how knowledge. It is this ability to recognise patterns which is the hallmark of Benner's (1984) expert model, in that practitioners form and develop paradigm cases from different patient episodes and approach patient care using previous concrete experiences. As practitioners build up this repertoire of paradigm cases, they reach the expert level. The ability of an expert nurse is to identify someone who may be experiencing pain but not showing overt signs, whereas perhaps a novice nurse would not see this due to lack of previous cases.

The importance of the 'knowing-that' (Ryle 2000) element of knowledge therefore takes on greater emphasis, particularly within the advanced practice debate, and yet knowing-that is not simply reading a textbook. Therefore, it would appear that the nature of advanced practice lies in the *integration* of knowing-how-why-what and knowing-that, and the advanced practitioner is the practical exemplar of this transition.

This leads to the question concerning *what* is needed for an individual practitioner to advance their practice. It would seem reasonable to suggest that within the context of advancing practice in pain management, the most appropriate model may consist of a process in which specialisation, expansion and advancement form the elements necessary to meet the requirements of advanced practice (American Nurses Association 1995; Hamric 2000). The reasons for this approach are that advancing practice is closely linked with the personal development of the individual (Fulbrook 1998) and is more focused on the 'how' of practice as opposed to the 'what' of practice (Rolfe 1998); the what is considered to be more aligned with advanced practice. This highlights the differences between advanced practice and advancing practice as well as basic nursing practice. Therefore, if this model is viewed as a pyramid of development, at its foundation is basic nursing practice and advanced practice at the apex, with progressional elements being specialisation, expansion and advancement (Figure 1.2).

Advancing practice is a continual developmental process which involves refining knowledge and skills to provide the precursor for advanced level practice in a systematic progression of individual professional and personal development. But advancing practice is more than simply acquiring experiential knowledge or academic qualifications at the behest of organisational or professional need. Advancing practice is also a process of continuing professional development utilising research, further education, leadership and clinical practice (Sams 1996; Wilson-Barnett *et al.* 2000), all of which culminate in a practitioner who is able to challenge and change professional boundaries, attain professional maturity and achieve higher levels of autonomy.

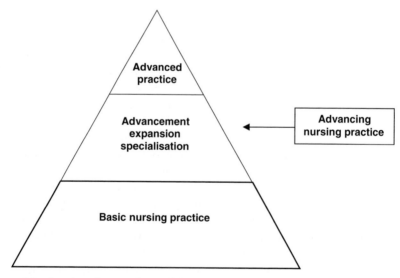

Figure 1.2   An advancing practice model of development.

What is important in terms of advancing practice is the *integration* of the different types of knowing and the understanding associated with this – the link between thinking and doing. Developing a mixture of knowing-how (practical knowing), knowing-why (theoretical knowing) and knowing-what (pattern recognition) leads to knowing-that. This is the choice of action determined by the practitioner's understanding of the situation. The situation or context of this will be illustrated by advanced (and advancing) practitioners working in the area of pain management.

The context of pain management: definitions and prevalence

Pain has been defined as 'whatever the experiencing person says it is and existing whenever he says it does' (McCaffery 1968). This is helpful as it emphasises believing the person and what they say about their pain. In 1979, the International Association for the Study of Pain (IASP) introduced the most widely used definition of pain and defined it as 'an unpleasant sensory and emotional experience associated with actual or potential tissue damage, or described in terms of such damage' (IASP Task Force on Taxonomy 1994). Whilst this is useful, it does not reflect the definition of chronic pain which McCaffery and Beebe (1989, p. 232) suggest is:

> Pain that has lasted 6 months or longer, is ongoing on a daily basis, is due to non-threatening causes, has not responded to currently available treatment methods, and may continue for the remainder of the patient's life.

This is but one definition and whilst the time periods may be different (perhaps 3 months), the essential tenet remains the same for many definitions. Pain can be viewed as a multidimensional experience which reflects emotional, sensory and cognitive elements. The experience of pain is complex and known to be influenced by a multitude of factors, including previous pain experiences, emotion, mood, culture, age and situation.

The inadequacies of the management of pain have been reported consistently for over 30 years (Marks & Sachar 1973; Fagerhaugh & Strauss 1977; Svensson *et al.* 2000, Kirou-Mauro *et al.* 2009). Despite improvements in acute pain management through the introduction of 'acute pain' teams and new technology such as patient-controlled analgesia, the management of acute pain following surgery has long been reported as problematic in the UK, USA and Europe (Clinical Standards Advisory Group 2000; Dolin *et al.* 2002; Visentin *et al.* 2005). In the community the picture is worse with chronic pain estimated to have a prevalence rate between 2 and 40% (Verhaak *et al.* 1998), and it is particularly problematic for those who are older or have difficulty communicating. In Europe it has been found that chronic pain of moderate-to-severe intensity occurs in 19% of adults, seriously affecting the quality of their social and working lives (Breivik *et al.* 2006). Many people with chronic pain often report poorer self-rated health, mental well-being and social functioning as well as greater levels of depression and work loss (Mallen *et al.* 2005).

The challenges of managing pain have been well documented, and it would be fair to say that whilst the management of acute pain and particularly that associated with surgery have shown radical improvement in recent years, many people continue to experience unrelieved chronic or persistent pain which is tremendously debilitating in terms of their function and quality of life. It is interesting that several of the contributors in this book chose to focus the development and delivery of a service for people whose pain was challenging to manage.

Advancing practice in pain management

The scene and context for this book have been set. Pain management is a challenging arena in which to practise, and those committed to making a difference face multiple challenges. So what would constitute advanced nursing practice in pain management? Despite an abundance of papers discussing 'advanced practice', few exist which specifically have discussed the contribution such nurses might make in pain management.

Using the British Nursing Index database and the search term 'advanced nursing' gives several hundred citations for each year over the past 10 years (see Table 1.2), yet adding the word 'pain' generates a fraction of results, on average less than 5%. The paucity of published papers in this area seems at odds with the prevalence pain management and in particular chronic pain. The management of chronic pain has traditionally been a poor relation to acute services and yet frequently provides an opportunity for nurses to take a lead in developing care and service delivery.

Despite the scarcity of studies and publications, there are some excellent examples of advanced nursing in pain management which cover a range of important areas. These range from how the role of the advanced practitioner can lessen the gap between

Table 1.2 British Nursing Index database and search terms 'advanced nursing' and 'pain' (1998–2008)

Year	Search term 'advanced nursing'	Addition of 'pain' as search term
1998–1999	704	36 (5.1%)
1999–2000	745	25 (3.4%)
2000–2001	766	25 (3.3%)
2001–2002	683	29 (4.2%)
2002–2003	578	28 (4.8%)
2003–2004	582	29 (5.0%)
2004–2005	611	25 (4.1%)
2005–2006	611	27 (4.4%)
2006–2007	585	28 (4.9%)
2007–2008	538	29 (5.4%)

knowledge and practice (Smith-Idell *et al.* 2007) to pushing boundaries of prescribing (Berry *et al.* 2007) and developing a telephone service for paediatric patients following spinal surgery (Carznecki *et al.* 2007).

Kohr and Sawhney (2005) conducted a web-based survey of how Canadian advanced nurse practitioners assisted patients in identifying their patient's pain management needs. One hundred sixteen nurses responded to the survey and 13% of these had a speciality practice in pain management. The survey identified known barriers to effective pain management, including insufficient education of nurse/physician teams, lack of patient education and lack of clear guidelines. They suggested that advanced nurse practitioner had a key role in supporting the use of practice guidelines and working collaboratively with colleagues, patients and their families. Many of the chapters in this book reflect such findings as they describe in detail the tortuous path undertaken to champion a service development. Much of the work has focused around the development of guidelines, algorithms and documentation to support new services as well as the myriad of other activities which are required to make it happen.

Before concluding this section it is important to bring in a few concluding thoughts on the attributes of advanced practice in the management of pain. There is no doubt that the highly valued skills relating to technical knowledge, physiology, psychology and sociology are central columns for the structure. There is a collection of other skills, sometimes less emphasised, which we believe are integral to the delivery of advanced care and would include the notion of being 'alongside' the patient. The ability to stay with someone as they experience pain, support them and give them a sense of your own sharing of their pain is an immensely skilful activity. The importance being *alongside* the person in pain is beautifully captured in an inspirational and sensitive book *Alongside the Patient in Pain* (Fordham & Dunn 1994). A recent paper exploring this concept for pain management makes an important connection between nurses' ability to share neurophysical empathy, which includes both somatosensory and emotional networks (Campbell-Yeo *et al.* 2008).

Bringing together advanced practice and pain management

In searching for generic features to pull together the diversity of activities which we believe informs the development of advanced practice in pain management, we drew on six important aspects which we wanted our authors to engage with when telling their stories. When describing how the service developed, it is easy to lose the essence of this rich and valuable experience, so we sought to shape the journey with subheadings which brought to light processes underlying their achievements. Making transparent this part of the journey permits others to draw on their achievements and 'test' this knowledge in a different setting. It also allows us to critically evaluate these contributions and in particular the 'advanced knowledge' contribution. Asking practitioners to reflect on their 'advanced contribution' recognises the importance of these practitioners having reflective skills (Glaze 2002) but does not necessarily suggest they are developed to full capacity. It was probably the hardest section of each chapter to write.

In Chapter 9, Dee Burrows describes how she led a multidisciplinary team in developing a pain management programme and associated services in the independent sector. This chapter captures a unique contribution as not only is it about a nurse consultant developing and leading a pain service but the context is outside the normal territory. It is a detailed account of the both the macro- and microconsiderations as well as an honest account of the struggles and successes, a blueprint for others.

Paul Bibby, in Chapter 8, similarly charts his own course outside the traditional structures of the NHS to describe how he set up a private company to provide a nurse-led clinic for patients with chronic neck (and shoulder) pain within the community. The chapter highlights the importance of policies influencing the provision of pain services and how commissioners, purchasers and those providing services have to work together. The importance of working across boundaries and not being inhibited to explore new boundaries are central to the narrative.

Conclusions

This opening chapter has attempted to put into context the nature of advanced and advancing practice by actively engaging in the ongoing debate about what constitutes advanced and advancing nursing practice within the context of pain management. There is a realisation that the accumulation of academic awards or length of service does not necessarily mean the advancement of practice. It is also evident that there exists a dichotomy as to what the true meanings of advanced and advancing practice actually are. Due to the lack of clarity over the two terms, we have adopted a working definition of advancing practice to illustrate the work presented here and to focus thinking around what the requirements for advancing practice are. The practitioner who is advancing their practice is able to challenge and change professional boundaries, attain professional maturity and achieve higher levels of autonomy.

The number of people experiencing unrelieved pain and the care available to them highlights the need for care which better meets their needs. The barriers impeding the effective delivery of care relate to the patients, the professionals and the organisations in which pain management takes place. The complexity of these situations requires professionals with vision, leadership, knowledge and skills, and a huge amount of tenacity. Each chapter highlights the problem and then provides a rich description of the journey to develop, deliver and evaluate a service. We believe these chapters capture an inspirational collection of practice, which highlights advanced and advancing care in pain management. We hope they will provide you with an opportunity to learn, reflect and be inspired.

References

American Nurses Association, 1995. *Nursing's Social Policy Statement*. Washington: American Nurses Association.

Atkins, S., Ersser, S.J., 2000. Education for advanced nursing practice: an evolving framework. *Journal of International Nursing Studies*, 37, 523–533.

Benner, P., 1984. *From Novice to Expert: Excellence and Power in Clinical Nursing Practice*, pp. 13–34. Menlo Park: Addison-Wesley.

Breivik, H., Collett, B., Ventafridda, V., Cohen, R., Gallacher, D., 2006. Survey of chronic pain in Europe: prevalence, impact on daily life, and treatment. *European Journal of Pain*, 10(4), 287–333.

Campbell-Yeo, M., Latimer, M., Johnston, C., 2008. The empathetic response in nurses who treat pain: a concept analysis. *Journal of Advanced Nursing*, 61(6), 711–719.

Castledine, G., 2004. The development of advanced nursing practice in the UK. In McGee, P., Castledine, G. (eds), *Advanced Nursing Practice*, 2nd edn, pp. 8–16. Oxford: Blackwell.

Christensen, M., 2009. Advancing practice in critical care: a model of knowledge integration. *Nursing in Critical Care*, 14(2), 86–94.

Clinical Standards Advisory Group, 2000. Services for patients with pain: a summary of the CSAG report on services for NHS patients with acute and chronic pain. Available at http://www.dh.gov.uk/en/Publicationsandstatistics/Publications/PublicationsPolicyAndGuidance/DH_4009217 [accessed 11 November 2008.

Davis, B., Hughes, A.M., 2002. Clarification of advanced nursing practice: characteristics and competencies. *Clinical Nurse Specialist*, 16, 147–152.

Dolin, S.J., Cashman, J.N., Bland, J.M., 2002. Effectiveness of acute postoperative pain management: evidence from published data. *British Journal of Anaesthesia*, 89(3), 409–423.

Dunn, L., 1997. A literature review of advanced clinical nursing practice in the United States of America. *Journal of Advanced Nursing*, 25, 814–819.

Fagerhaugh, S.H., Strauss, A., 1977. *Politics of Pain Management*. Reading, MA: Addison-Wesley.

Fordham, M., Dunn, V., 1994. *Alongside the Patient in Pain: Holistic Care and Nursing Practice*. London: Balliere Tindall.

Fulbrook, P., 1998. Advanced practice: the 'advanced practitioner' perspective. In Rolfe, G., Fulbrook, P. (eds), *Advanced Nursing Practice*, pp. 83–102. Oxford: Butterworth-Heinemann.

Hamric, A.B., 2000. A definition of advanced nursing practice. In Hamric, A.B., Spross, J.A., Hanson, C.M.. (eds), *Advanced Nursing Practice: An Integrative Approach*, 2nd edn, pp. 53–74. Philadelphia: W.B. Saunders.

International Council of Nurses, 2006. *Definition and Characteristics of the Role*. Geneva: ICN.

Jamieson, L., Mosel-Williams, L., Dwyer, T., 2002. The need for an advanced nursing practice role for Australian adult critical care settings. *Australian Critical Care*, 15(4), 139–145.

Jenkins, R.L., White, P., 2001. Telehealth advancing nursing practice. *Nursing Outlook,* 49(2), 100–105.

Jackson, P.L., Kennedy, C., Slaughter, R., 2003. Employment characteristics of recent PNP graduates. *Journal of Pediatric Health Care*, 17(3), 133–139.

Kirou-Mauro, A.M., Hird, A., Wong, J., Sinclair, E., Barnes, E.A., Tsao, M., Danjoux, C., Chow, E., 2009. Has pain management in cancer patients with bone metastases improved? A seven-year review at an outpatient palliative radiotherapy clinic. *Journal of Pain and Symptom Management*, 37(1), 77–84.

Mallen, C., Peat, G., Thomas, E., Croft, P., 2005. Severely disabling chronic pain in young adults: prevalence from a population-based postal survey in North Staffordshire. *BMC Musculoskeletal Disorders*, 6, 42.

Marks, R., Sachar, E., 1973. Undertreatment of medical in-patients with narcotic analgesics. *Annals of Internal Medicine*, 78(2), 173–181.

McCaffery, M., 1968. *Nursing Practice Theories Related to Cognition, Bodily Pain and Non-Environment Interactions*. Los Angeles, CA: University of California.

McCaffery, M., Beebe, A., 1989. *Pain: Clinical Manual for Nursing Practice*. St. Louis, MO: CV Mosby.

McGee, P., Castledine, G., 2003. A definition of advanced practice for the UK. In McGee, P., Castledine, G. (eds), *Advanced Nursing Practice*, 2nd edn, pp. 17–30. Oxford: Blackwell Publishing.

H. Merskey and N. Bogduk, 1994. Classification of chronic pain. In H. Merskey and N. Bogduk, (eds), *Part III: pain terms, a current list with definitions and notes on usage. IASP task force on taxonomy*, pp. 209–214. Seattle: IASP Press.

Por, J., 2008. A critical engagement with the concept of advancing nursing practice. *Journal of Nursing Management*, 16, 84–90.

Rolfe, G., 1998. Education for the advanced practitioner. In Rolfe, G., Fulbrook, P. (eds), *Advanced Nursing Practice*, pp. 271–280. Oxford: Butterworth-Heinemann.

Royal College of Nursing, 2003. *Nurse Practitioners: An RCN Guide to the Nurse Practitioner Role, Competencies and Programme Accreditation*. London: RCN.

Ryle, G., 2000. *The Concept of Mind*. London: Penguin Books.

Sams, D., 1996. Developing advanced nursing practice. *British Journal of Community Health Nursing*, 1, 355–361.

Scholes, J., 2006. *Developing Expertise in Critical Care Nursing*. Oxford: Blackwell Publishing.

Schon, D.A., 1983. *The Reflective Practitioner: How Professionals Think in Action*. London: Ashgate.

Thompson, D.R., Watson, R., 2003. Advanced nursing practice: What is it? *International Journal of Nursing Practice*, 9, 129–130.

United Kingdom Central Council (UKCC), 1996. *PREP — The Nature of Advanced Practice. An Interim Report*. London: UKCC.

Verhaak, P.M., Kerssens, J.J., Dekker, J., Sorbi, M.J., Bensing, J.M., 1998. Prevalence of chronic benign pain disorder among adults: a review of the literature. *Pain*, 77, 231–239.

Visentin, M., Zanolin, E., Trentin, L., Sartori, S., de Marco, R., 2005. Prevalence and treatment of pain in adults admitted to Italian hospitals. *European Journal of Pain*, 9(1),61–67.

Wilson-Barnett, J., Barriball, L.K., Reynolds, H., Jowett, S., Ryrie, I., 2000. Recognising advancing nursing practice: evidence from two observational studies. *International Journal of Nursing Studies*, 37, 389–400.

Woods, L.P., 1999. The contingent nature of advanced nursing practice. *Journal of Advanced Nursing*, 30(1), 121–128.

Chapter 2
Nurse-led femoral nerve block service for patients with fractured neck of femur

Mandy Layzell

Introduction

Fractures of the hip are relatively common amongst older people and can have serious consequences, with a mortality rate of 10% at 1 month after a fall, 20% at 4 months and 30% at 1 year (Parker & Johansen 2006). Many of those who recover suffer a loss in mobility and independence. The average age for this group of patients is over 80 years and the majority (75%) are female. Many of these patients have significant comorbidities and are often taking numerous medications that may delay surgery and their recovery. In addition to a hip fracture, they often present in accident and emergency with acute medical problems such as chest or urine infections or heart failure, which may well have been the cause of the fall. This group of patients are likely to be malnourished on admission and show a rapid deterioration in nutritional status during admission (Nematy *et al*. 2006).

Hip fractures account for 87% of the total cost of all fragility fractures, making them the most expensive fractures associated with osteoporosis. In 2005–2006, 68 416 patients with a fractured neck of femur were operated on in England, with an average length of hospital stay of 25.7 days at a cost to the NHS of at least £384 million (Institute for Innovation and Improvement 2006). The incidence of hip fractures worldwide in 1990 was 1.26 million and with the projected increase in the elderly population, the number is predicted to be 2.6 million in 2025 and 4.5 million by 2050 (Gullberg *et al*. 1997). Locally the number of patients admitted to the trust with fractured neck of femur in 2008 was in excess of 900, which is possibly the highest in the UK.

The Royal College of Physicians' guidelines *Fractured Neck of Femur: Prevention and Management* recommend that patients should be operated on within 24 hours; in practice, this is often hard to achieve for a variety of reasons. For example, some patients are unwell and need medical investigation and intervention; often these patients are delayed or cancelled due to more serious admissions taking priority, and also due to lack of theatre sessions and available staff. Recent evidence states that a delay beyond 48 hours to operation is associated with a higher risk of mortality and an increase in length of post-operative stay (Bottle & Aylin 2006). Williams and Jester (2005) recommend that patients whose surgery is delayed should receive intensive nursing care in an attempt to optimise their condition. This includes adequate pain control, fluid and oxygen resuscitation, and adequate pressure area care to ensure they are as 'fit' as possible for surgery.

Improving pain relief and relieving suffering is at the core of nursing, and working as a lead nurse for acute pain puts me in a strong position for highlighting areas of need and changing practice. I am fortunate to work in a trust which acknowledges the value of specialist nurses and will support them to embrace innovation to enhance the patient's experience and provide best practice. Patients awaiting theatre for hip fixation require basic nursing care such as pain relief, prevention of pressure sores and nutrition. Inadequate pain management prevents all of these being performed effectively; therefore, improving pain management is paramount to ensure these patients are in optimum condition prior to surgery. This chapter describes how I have led a team of nurses in implementing a service to improve pain relief and aid basic nursing care for patients following hip fracture.

Pain control

Pain is one of the factors that trigger the injury response, resulting in metabolic, endocrine and water and electrolyte changes that may have an adverse effect on recovery, and current evidence indicates that effective pain control is capable of modifying these responses (Vickers 2007). Fractures cause significant pain, which can be exacerbated by movement, and so for patients with a fractured neck of femur, pain control in the immediate post-trauma period can be difficult to manage effectively. While the emergency management of major trauma has been extensively analysed in the last few years, trauma analgesia has received comparatively little attention. Reluctance to deliver adequate pain relief in the acute stage of trauma originates, at least in part, from a widely held belief that analgesia may precipitate or disguise cardiorespiratory deterioration (Coleman 2003). In reality, current evidence shows that uncontrolled pain may actually harm patients by impairing cardiac, pulmonary and endocrine functioning (Macintyre & Schug 2007).

A growing body of research supports the link between serious post-operative complications such as deep vein thrombosis, infections, sepsis, paralytic ileus, acute renal failure and uncontrolled pain (Australian and New Zealand College of Anaesthetists and Faculty of Pain Medicine 2005). In addition, pain interferes with sleep, impairs immune functioning and lowers the quality of life for the patient (Arnstein 2002). The physiological changes that result from pain and injury are a result of activation of both the peripheral and the central nervous systems. Trauma and injury induce a complex 'stress response' characterised by hormonal changes and an inflammatory response leading to malaise, hyperthermia and immunosuppression. Effective analgesia is capable of modifying many of the pathophysiological responses, preventing or reducing complications and assisting recovery. Regular pain assessment and evaluation of effect are vital by nursing staff to ensure that patients do not experience severe pain and side effects from analgesia.

Under-treated pain

The assessment of pain in others is notoriously difficult, but it is the professional responsibility of the nurse to carry out an assessment. Older people form the population most at risk of having their pain inadequately assessed, and this is especially so for those with dementia (Weiner & Hanlon 2001). This group have a higher risk of complications due to unrelieved or under-treated pain and so they are particularly likely to benefit from effective pain management. However, a number of factors may combine to make control of pain more difficult than in a younger patient (Rowbotham & Macintyre 2003). These include the following:

- Coexistent diseases and concurrent medications, putting them at risk from drug–drug and disease–drug interactions;
- Diminished functional status and physiological reserve;
- Age-related changes in pharmacodynamics and pharmacokinetics;
- Altered pain responses;
- Difficulties in the assessment of pain, including problems related to cognitive impairment and communication.

Pharmacokinetics

The pharmacokinetics (absorption, distribution, metabolism and excretion) of many drugs are altered in the elderly; these changes are generally attributable to ageing alone but may be compounded by the higher incidence of degenerative and other concurrent diseases. The physiological changes can vary widely between individuals, with the most significant being related to cardiac output and renal function. In addition, changes in liver function and protein binding may have some effect.

Pharmacodynamics

It is not fully understood how these age-related changes in response to drugs occur. Studies indicate that in the elderly population, sensitivity of the brain to opioids is increased by about 50%; it is uncertain if this is due to alterations in the number and/or function of opioid receptors in the central nervous system, or to other factors (Australian and New Zealand College of Anaesthetists and Faculty of Pain Medicine 2005).

Changes in pain perception

The widespread belief that elderly patients experience less pain lacks scientific support. In general, in the nervous system of the elderly person, there are extensive alterations in structure, neurochemistry and function of both the peripheral and central nervous systems. Therefore, there may be changes in the way that pain is processed, including impairment of the pain inhibitory system (Australian and New Zealand College of Anaesthetists and Faculty of Pain Medicine 2005).

Assessment of pain

Older people form the population most at risk of having their pain inadequately assessed, and this is especially so for those with dementia. Pain is a personal experience and self-reporting of pain is considered to be the best approach to pain assessment. However, undetected pain in this group of patients is a significant problem for a number of reasons. These include differences in reporting pain (Rowbotham & Macintyre 2003), disparity in the perception of pain between patients and caregivers (Whipple *et al.* 1995), insufficient education and/or training for nursing staff (Cohen Mansfield & Creedon 2002), cognitive impairment and difficulties in measurement (Morrison & Siu 2000) and non-use of pain assessment tools (McAuliffe *et al.* 2009). In addition, psychological and cultural factors, such as fear, anxiety, depression, the implication of the traumatic event, loss of independence, feelings of isolation, the quality of social support available, and family, will all affect reporting of pain and ultimately assessment and management.

Analgesic drugs and the elderly

The management of acute pain involves the use of systemic opioids, paracetamol and non-steroidal anti-inflammatory drugs (NSAIDs). This multimodal approach – a combination of two or more analgesic modalities with differing analgesic mechanisms – is considered to be best practice to enhance analgesia and reduce side effects (Myles & Power 2007). Whilst paracetamol is a relatively safe and effective adjunct for pain relief, it will not give sufficient relief alone for a fracture. The use of NSAIDs in this group of patients significantly increases the risk of complications such as upper gastrointestinal haemorrhage and renal failure (Pirmohamed *et al.* 2004). Opioids are effective analgesics, but effective and safe doses are difficult to titrate in the elderly due to the large inter-patient variability. Elderly patients generally do appear to require less opioid than younger patients; therefore, careful titration at appropriate dose intervals is required to prevent undesirable side effects. In practice, many physicians are reluctant to prescribe opioid analgesics to elderly patients and nursing staff are often hesitant to administer for fear of side effects (Pasero & McCaffrey 1996, 1997a, b). Opioid use and under-treated pain have been shown to increase the incidence of delirium (Morrison *et al.* 2003a) and slow post-operative mobilisation and recovery (Morrison *et al.* 2003b).

Adequate pain relief on general wards is dependent on the assessment of pain and administration of analgesia by nursing staff. Willson (2000) conducted a study looking at factors which affected the administration of analgesia to patients following a repair of a fractured hip. She identified that the decision made by nurses to administer analgesia is not simply a matter of education and adherence to the drug prescription, but a consequence of an interplay of a number of factors. These include organisation of the ward, demands made by the shift, concerns over the use of opioid analgesia and the way in which information is communicated. Willson (2000) found that in some cases nurses were prepared to accept a more alert patient who was able to participate in rehabilitation in place of adequate pain relief.

Many of the patients who are admitted with a fractured hip often have other comorbidities which restrict the use of the range of drugs normally used for acute pain relief, such as NSAIDs; this creates further challenges to pain management. Therefore, pain relief, which is long-lasting, does not cause any significant side effects and does not require extra work for the ward nursing staff, which is appealing. McQuay and Moore (1998) reported that the use of local anaesthetic has a perceived advantage because it can deliver complete pain relief by interrupting pain transmission from a localised area, thereby avoiding generalised adverse drug effects from opioids and NSAIDs.

Femoral nerve block

Boyd *et al*. (2006) describe regional analgesia techniques as providing superior postoperative analgesia, higher levels of patient's satisfaction and reduced morbidity and mortality in patients with certain comorbid conditions. Local anaesthetic nerve blocks either as a single shot or continuous infusion technique are, therefore, particularly suited to elderly patients. Studies suggest that peripheral nerve blocks may have a role to play in the perioperative management of pain (Haddad & Williams 1995; Fletcher *et al*. 2003), but little is known about their specific value in the pre-operative period. Pre-operative nerve blocks are recommended by the New Zealand Guidelines Group (2003) as part of the acute management for patients with hip fracture. An appropriate, safe and easily executed nerve block for fractured neck of femur is a femoral nerve block (FNB). The technique involves identification of the femoral nerve in the groin with the use of a nerve stimulator and injection of local anaesthetic solution in close proximity to the femoral and adjacent nerves. The local anaesthetic tracks along the femoral sheath to anaesthetise the femoral, obturator, lateral femoral cutaneous nerve of the thigh and the lower cords of the lumbar plexus (Hurley 2004), thus reducing the pain experienced for patients who have a hip fracture.

Benefits of FNB

Once familiar with the technique, FNB is a relatively simple procedure to perform, with good evidence to suggest that the onset of analgesia is fast and effective and the analgesic effect can last between 6 and 8 hours. In some cases analgesia may be present for up to 24 hours (Harper 2001). There is some evidence that an FNB may give better analgesia for lower, inter-trochanteric fractures than for higher cervical fractures, but significant improvement in pain scores are seen for both types (Fletcher *et al*. 2003). Use of local anaesthetic blocks perioperatively has been associated with a reduction in pain and fewer complications post-operatively (Boyd *et al.* 2006). In addition, improved pain relief will allow patients to move around the bed more easily, therefore reducing the risk of developing pressure sores, and patients will be able to sit up to eat and drink to ensure adequate nutrition.

Risks of FNB

Published evidence suggests that FNB carries a very low risk of adverse events (Haddad & Williams 1995; Auory *et al.* 1997; Fletcher *et al.* 2003); the most likely risks include haematoma, nerve damage, infection and intravascular injection with toxicity. These are complications shared by all regional blocks and can be minimised by the use of careful technique, strict exclusion criteria (Table 2.1) and the use of levobupivacaine (rather than bupivacaine). Levobupivacaine carries lower risk of the central nervous system and cardiovascular system toxicity and may cause shorter motor blockade and longer sensory blockade (Australian and New Zealand College of Anaesthetists and Faculty of Pain Medicine 2005).

Rationale for a nurse-led service

New opportunities have arisen for nurses to develop and lead new services with the introduction of specialist and advanced nursing roles and the reduction in junior doctors' hours. Traditionally, doctors working in anaesthesia or Accident and Emergency (A/E)

Table 2.1   Contraindications for performing a femoral nerve block (FNB)

Contraindications for FNB
Absolute
Patient refusal
Anticoagulant therapy
Clotting disorders (International Normalising Ration (INR) >1.5 or platelets <80)
Established allergy to local anaesthetics
Infection at injection site
Previous femoral vascular surgery
Anatomy precluding clear identification of landmarks
Relative
Respiratory rate <10
Systolic BP <90 mm Hg
Patient agitated/unable to cooperate
Acutely ill (septic, severe heart failure, myocardial infarction, acute respiratory failure)

were taught how to perform an FNB and if the doctor had time the patient would be given a block before being transferred to the general ward. Local audit data and feedback from nursing staff revealed that pain management for this group of patients was inadequate and patients often experienced excruciating pain, very few received a nerve block in A/E. Consideration was given to the possibility of training the junior doctors, but these doctors are transient in the hospital and the time and resources required to train and monitor such a group of doctors in giving an effective FNB service was not a feasible undertaking. In addition, the A/E doctors or on-call anaesthetists have duties which take priority over what is a potentially time-consuming technique. Specialist nurses working in acute pain teams are ideally placed to take on the training and develop skills to deliver an FNB block service for patients with fractured neck of femur.

Developing the service

Previous trust audit data highlighted that pain management for patients admitted following trauma was problematic, in particular those patients admitted following a fall and fracturing their neck of femur. Over recent years we introduced a pre-printed analgesia label which was attached to the drug chart to ensure that all trauma and surgical patients received a range of analgesics to manage acute pain and deal with any side effects (Layzell 2005). Unfortunately, systemic analgesia alone is unlikely to give effective pain relief during movement, and as this group of patients are often frail, the likelihood of serious side effects is quite high. The complexity of patient needs and the gap in pain provision was challenging. It was evident that there was an opportunity for a nurse-led service for patients with fractured neck of femur who are likely to wait for surgery. Ideally, patients should be operated on within 48 hours; over the last year in the trust, 59–88% of patients were operated on within this time period.

Protocol development and training

Implementing change in services requires substantial effort and needs to be driven by a motivated and enthusiastic team. As lead nurse for the team I was responsible for discussing with my two other colleagues what would be involved and the training required to develop and implement this new service. I had to make sure they were aware that we would increase our workload quite substantially and that we may have to adjust our working hours to ensure we could complete the supervised blocks. In addition, they needed to be willing to take on the training, advance their knowledge and level of practice to a higher level. The team were keen to take on this challenge of learning advanced skills and push forward into new arenas of health care that would ultimately benefit this group of vulnerable patients. The team would integrate this extra work into their normal working day, and at this stage there was no request for additional nursing staff.

Prior to the implementation of the FNB service, it was essential to develop a protocol and gain approval by the hospital executive committee, physicians, nursing staff and managers. Initially, a presentation to the hospital executive committee was made and approval was given for us to run a 12-month pilot project. As this service was to be completely nurse-led, it was important to acknowledge professional responsibility and accountability. The Nursing and Midwifery Council (NMC) (2008) requires that 'care should be delivered on the best available evidence or best practice' and that individual practitioners must have 'the knowledge and skills for safe and effective practice when working without direct supervision'. I ensured that these essential requirements were built into the protocol. Letters were sent out explaining our proposal to consultants, ward sisters and relevant mangers, and an invitation to respond to our proposal. We did anticipate that there would be some objections but surprisingly we had unanimous approval and encouragement to set up the service. All health care workers are aware of the difficulties with managing pain in this group of patients and if an intervention is likely to improve pain relief and outcome then there is little to object to.

The most time-consuming part of the service development was steering the protocol through the relevant hospital policy groups. The protocol incorporated a training manual complete with explanations of the procedure, equipment required, a knowledge and skills framework, patient information sheet, patient group directives for local anaesthetics and audit data collection process. Only nurses working in the acute pain team were eligible to train and provide this service. We did anticipate that once we had completed the pilot project we could expand the training to the trauma nurse practitioners so that we could extend the service to weekends.

Patient information sheet

Information is an important part of the patient journey and central to the overall quality of each patient's experience of the NHS. The leaflet was designed to allow patients to make an informed consent so that they, or their carers, could make a rational decision on whether they wanted a nerve block. The leaflet discusses the following:

- Problems and risks with some painkillers;
- Information about how the block is performed and by whom;
- How long the block lasts;
- Benefits and risks associated with the FNB.

The leaflet was vetted by the Patient Advisory Liaison Service and the hospital readership panel before agreement was given. For further information on developing patient information leaflets, go to www.nhsidentity.nhs.uk/patientinformationtoolkit/patientinfotoolkit.pdf.

Patient group directions

To perform the nerve block it is necessary for lidocaine to be used to numb the skin in the groin and for levobupivacaine to be injected in close proximity to the femoral nerve to produce pain relief. As this procedure was to be performed independently by the nurses without medical input, it was necessary to develop patient group directions (PGDs) for both of these drugs. PGDs allow a nurse who is authorised to administer a medicine to a specific group of patients. They are useful in situations where a limited range of indications apply to a large number of patients. They offer an advantage for patient care without compromising safety and are consistent with appropriate professional relationships and accountability. In order for a PGD to be approved, it must be agreed and signed for by a doctor and pharmacist, and relevant heads of departments within the local trust. This document is then reviewed biannually.

Data collection and evaluation of the service

The trust agreed to allow the service to run as a 12-month pilot project, extending this service was subjected to review by the hospital executive committee after the pilot project had been completed. To demonstrate safety and effectiveness of the service it was necessary to perform a clinical audit. Due to staff numbers and hours of work it was not feasible to collect a large amount of data; so for the data to be accurate and meaningful, we had to decide exactly what data we could realistically collect. An example is given below:

- Date and time of admission.
- Date and time of nerve block.
- Pain scores pre- and post-block – the subjective nature of pain was assessed using a numerical verbal pain score, with 0 being no pain and 10 being the worst pain experienced.
- Passive hip flexion using a goniometer – to provide a measurement of the impact of pain on function we recorded pre- and post-block hip flexion. This requires two members of staff, one person will lift the affected leg to the point of pain and the other person will record the measurement.
- Analgesia uses 8 hours pre- and post-block.
- Complications – such as arterial puncture, intravascular injection, signs of toxicity and collapse.

Training

As this service was to be completely nurse-led, it was necessary for the team to undergo training in taking consent for patients with and without capacity, IV cannulation and advanced resuscitation skills. In addition, training was required in the administration of local anaesthetic under a PGD. Named anaesthetists competent in the technique and equipment carried out the training and assessment. Competency, as agreed by the local trust, was based around a knowledge and skills framework and successful completion of ten supervised blocks. Review of skills was performed by the Acute Pain Team's clinical lead, initially monthly for 4 months and then six monthly.

Problems encountered with the training

This new service required the nurses in the team to work at an advanced nursing level by working independently and utilising skills of assessment, treatment, evaluation and data collection. The protocol provided the team with the background knowledge required to assess suitable patients, instructions how to perform the nerve block competently and deal with complications if they arose. In practice, there are likely to be situations which do not neatly fit into the protocol guidelines, and in the early days there were some clinical situations encountered which made the assessment criteria unclear and clarification from a medical colleague had to be sought. Physical examination is not normally part of a nurse's scope of practice, and time and effort was required to become familiar with examination to identify the relevant anatomy to establish the presence of the femoral artery. For logistical reasons the blocks would have to be performed single-handed or not at all. This was possible to do safely but would require very careful planning, considerable skill and dexterity. Traditionally, the procedure is performed with two people, one person to perform the block and an assistant to operate the specialised electronic equipment to locate the femoral nerve.

The biggest problem encountered with the training was the unpredictability of when these patients would present in A/E or transfer to the ward. Daily admissions range from 0 to 5 at anytime of the day or night, and as the acute pain team (APT) work only Monday to Friday 8 a.m. till 4 p.m., patients were missed. In order to provide consistency in teaching and technique, two anaesthetists carried out the training; this created another problem. Time was spent waiting for the anaesthetist to be free to supervise the block. Some members of the team worked part-time hours, which meant that it took several weeks to supervise, performing the necessary number of blocks. The team also had to ensure that other areas of their day-to-day role were not neglected and so consequently the pressures from increased activity were high. Due to the problems encountered, this initial training took several weeks.

Challenges in implementing a new service

It is well reported that pain is under-recognised and under-treated in older people. Pain management does not feature as a government target but does fit into several government policies. The *National Service Framework for Older People* was published in 2001 (Department of Health 2001) and states that the appropriate management of pain is essential to ensure the dignity and well-being of older people. Caring for frail older people is core business in the NHS and the White Paper 'Our health, our care, our say', which creates the opportunity to align the planning, commissioning and delivery of health and care for frail older people. The paper 'Focus on: fractured neck of femur' (NHS Institute for Innovation and Improvement 2006) emphasises on delivering high-quality, evidence-based delivery of services and suggests ways to improve services. Pain management is an essential component of the pathway as acknowledged in the New Zealand's *Best Practice Evidence-Based Guidelines*. These guidelines recommend the use of local analgesic nerve blocks in the pre-operative period to reduce the need for parenteral or oral analgesia whilst waiting for surgery. In my trust we have the second highest number of patients admitted with fractured neck of femur in the UK; therefore, this group of patients represent a large proportion of patients nursed on acute wards. I am frequently asked by nursing staff to help with pain management for these patients, and as previously discussed, analgesia and potential side effects are an area of concern. These documents provided me with evidence to support the implementation of a new service to improve pain management for this group of patients.

Introducing new services into the cash-conscious NHS requires careful planning, drive, commitment and determination. In the early planning stages I discussed with the team the possibility of incorporating the extra work generated from performing blocks into our normal working day. If we could achieve this we knew that our proposal would have a stronger case for service development and an increased possibility of the trust agreeing to run a pilot study. We anticipated that there would probably be around three blocks per day to do, and as most days there would be two members of staff working we felt we could integrate these into our daily workload. We were also fortunate to be offered free equipment for 1 year by a manufacturing company which already provided the hospital with nerve block needles. This meant that the only cost for the procedure would be for drugs, disposable items and paperwork, costing around £5.00 per patient. As we were not looking for additional staff or a large amount of money to get the service up and running, we did not develop a business plan. Instead a proposal was put forward to the hospital executive committee for approval. It can be difficult to introduce new services into the NHS unless they will have an effect on local trusts objectives or national targets, or procedures which have been approved by National Institute for Health and Clinical Excellence (NICE). In some cases proving that a service can work safely, efficiently and show improvements in patient care and experience, securing additional funding can be the best approach. Individual trusts work in very different ways and my past experience in my trust informed me that this approach is the way forward in this situation.

Evaluation of the 1-year pilot study

To demonstrate safety and effectiveness of the service it was necessary to perform a clinical audit. As previously mentioned, only basic audit data were collected due to limited time available by the nurses. During the pilot project a total of 807 patients were admitted to the hospital with a fractured neck of femur and the team were able to perform a block on 224 patients (Table 2.2). Data were recorded only if the patient received a nerve block; those who either refused or were not suitable for a block or who went to theatre on day of admission were not included in the database.

Table 2.2 Monthly admissions of patients with fractured neck of femur (#NOF) and the number of blocks performed

	Jan	Feb	Mar	Apr	May	Jun	July	Aug	Sep	Oct	Nov	Dec
#NOF admitted	66	53	74	70	72	77	72	68	69	66	63	57
Blocks performed	16	12	10	12	13	31	27	21	16	21	25	20

Table 2.3   Response time to performing FNB ($n = 224$)

	Number and percentage of patients
Block performed on day of admission	99 (44%)
Block performed within 24 hours	59 (26%)
Block performed >24 hours	64 (29%)
Incomplete data	2 (<1%)

Ideally, an FNB is best performed on admission to A/E. However, the team only work weekdays and between 8 a.m. and 4 p.m. In spite of this, approximately 70% of patients received a block within 24 hours of admission to hospital (Table 2.3).

The subjective nature of pain was assessed using a numerical verbal pain score, with 0 being no pain and 10 being the worst pain experienced. Scores were collected before the block was performed and 2 hours after. As a proportion of patients were likely to have communication difficulties if the patient could not give a pain score, we also recorded this. Around a third of the patients were not able to give a valid pain score, but of those that could we found that an average 3-point reduction on the 0–10 scale could be achieved (Figure 2.1).

To provide a measurement of the impact of pain on function we assessed the pain-free range of passive hip flexion pre-block and again 2 hours post-block as performed in the study by Candal-Couto *et al.* (2005). This requires two members of staff, one person will lift the affected leg to the point of pain whilst the other person will measure the angle. We were able to show that following the nerve block patients were able to tolerate an average of 20° increased passive hip flexion (Figure 2.2).

In addition to pain scores and passive hip flexion, we collected data on analgesia requirements 8 hours before and after the block. Generally a reduction in opioid use was demonstrated, but we felt this was not an accurate record of patient requirement as patients were totally dependent on firstly being able to ask the ward nursing staff for oral analgesia, and secondly the ward nurses being free to administer analgesia. Regarding the safety aspect of the specialist nurses performing these blocks in general

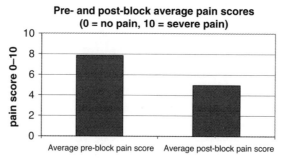

Figure 2.1   Average pre-block and 2 hours post-block pain scores.

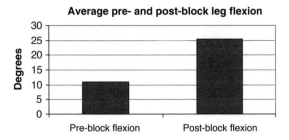

Figure 2.2   Average pre-block leg flexion and flexion 2 hours post-block.

wards, only one accidental arterial stab occurred; no other adverse events or incidence of complications was observed.

Service feedback from staff

To support the audit data a questionnaire was given randomly to staff involved in the care of this group of patients, including physiotherapists and medical and nursing staff. They were asked their opinion on whether they felt that the FNB provided pain relief and if it allowed the patients to move, eat and sleep more easily. Staff felt that patients who had had a block appeared to have less pain and improvements in mobility (in bed), nutrition and sleep (Layzell 2009).

Service feedback from patients

As yet we have not performed any further routine patient audit, although many will thank us for performing the nerve block as their pain is greatly reduced whilst they wait for theatre. One patient provided us with a quote for the local newspaper:

> I was in a lot of pain and it wasn't pleasant – after the nerve block, I felt as though my whole leg was made of wood, but I had no more pain! It was very effective and lasted about 24 hours. If you're in pain and somebody gets shot of it for you, you're very grateful.

Justifying the advanced nursing contribution

The relief from pain is a basic human right, and for nurses and health care workers caring for patients in pain is an important and often overlooked part of everyday care. The role of the nurse has changed over recent years with the introduction of specialist roles, reduction in junior doctors' hours and increase in demands on the NHS to provide better access and services. Specialist clinical roles have contributed enormously to improving services, and advanced practice roles have taken this one step further. I feel that my involvement in developing and leading the FNB service is a good example of advanced nursing practice for the following reasons.

The NMC (2006) describe advanced nursing practitioners as 'highly experienced, knowledgeable and educated members of the care team who are able to diagnose and treat the patients' health care needs'. The FNB service was developed to address some of the difficulties in managing pain for patients who have fractured their neck of femur and are waiting for surgery. Patients are referred to us either by medical or nursing staff in A/E or on the wards or by liaising with the specialist trauma nurses. Prior to performing the block, it is essential to assess the suitability of the patients from medical notes and most importantly that the patient is happy to consent to having a block. Written patient information and verbal explanations are given prior to obtaining informed written consent from the patient or carers, if necessary. Many of the patients admitted have some degree of cognitive impairment or transient confusion. In these cases Form 4 consent is used and where possible agreement from a partner or carer or in some circumstances a second opinion from one of the medical staff responsible for the care of the patient in hospital.

Performing the FNBs requires some dexterity. Traditionally, two people would be required, one to locate the nerve using specialist catheter and an assistant to operate the nerve stimulator. We presumed that most of the time we would be working on our own, so from the outset we were taught to perform the block single-handed, which required some familiarity and practice with the procedure to become competent; this has become easier with time, and the time to perform the block has reduced substantially from the earlier blocks performed. Local anaesthetics are administered under a local trust PGD and doses are given according to the patient's weight.

It is essential that the appropriate members of the health care team are informed and so a sticker is placed in the medical notes detailing procedure, a record is made on the patients drug chart and a verbal handover of the procedure is given to the nurse caring for the patient. In addition, a set of observations are recorded 10 minutes post-block and a checklist for possible complications and management advice for nursing staff is left on the patient's observation chart. We will then follow up the patient 2 hours post-block and again the next day to collect audit data. As team leader I am responsible for ensuring that the service is run safely. I will provide support and supervision for my colleagues in the team and discuss any issues that are raising concern. I regularly review audit data we collect to ensure that the procedure is performed safely and that patients are benefiting, and progress is disseminated to management and specialist committee members. In addition, I am responsible for ensuring that the relevant documentation is up to date and evidence-based.

There are several differences in the way that I am working as an advanced nurse compared to a doctor. Firstly, I will obtain informed consent from the patient and leave them with a copy of the consent form and a patient information sheet with my contact details included. Generally I have not seen a doctor take written consent for this procedure or provide written information. Doctors require the assistance of a nurse to provide them with the necessary equipment, position the patient, record observations, assist with the nerve block and dispose of the equipment after the procedure. I will do all of this alone. And finally, I will ensure that accurate records are left in the patient's medical notes and that nurses have appropriate guidance on action to take if complications occur. Doctors are often not as thorough as this. In addition, I will collect information for audit and do a follow-up visit myself, if the block has been performed in A/E. Doctors are unlikely to do a follow-up visit with the patient and will not collect any audit data.

For nurses to work at an advanced level it is necessary to have a higher level of knowledge and skills. In addition, it is essential that there are several other key components. There has to be a clear and evidence-based need for change in practice and evidence that current practice is not addressing this need; in this case audit data indicated a problem with pain management. The driver(s) for change has to be motivated and committed in their quest for service improvement, and also be prepared to work differently, by learning new skills. The advanced practitioner needs to be aware of local and national policies which affect health care and can assist in developing new services, such as evidence-based guidelines for the specific patient groups and PGDs to enable nurses to administer drugs without a doctor's prescription. And finally, the success of implementing such a service is dependent on hospital management, allowing the service development to exist. If I had not been able to secure this agreement in the early stages, it would not have been possible for me, and my colleagues, to work at an advanced level. In summary, as an advanced nurse I am able to provide a complete package of care for the patient and I am able to evaluate the effectiveness and safety of the procedure.

Conclusions

Pain management following a fractured neck of femur can be difficult to manage with traditional analgesics; in addition to this, problems exist with nurse's assessment of pain, particularly in patients with cognitive impairment. As the elderly population increases and the number of falls and fractures increase, new approaches to pain management are vital. Experienced nurses working in pain management are ideally placed to develop and lead new services and enhance their skills with the ultimate aim to improve pain management and relieve suffering for this group of patients. This chapter has discussed the vision of a team willing to face today's challenges in the NHS and embrace innovative ways of working. It has been demonstrated that it is possible to establish an entirely nurse-led service for performing FNB on pre-operative patients admitted with fractured neck of femur.

I hope that this work will inspire other teams around the UK to follow our example and help to relieve the suffering and improve the outcome for a significant group of vulnerable patients. Providing this service in the trust has been rewarding, firstly because patients are so grateful and impressed that someone is showing an interest in their pain relief. Previously, most of these patients suffered severe pain on movement, severely restricting sitting up to eat or drink. We have witnessed these patients in severe pain and unable to move, have performed a block and after 2 hours return to check the patient, have seen them sitting up in bed, eating, drinking, more comfortable and in some cases virtually pain free. To see this is tremendously satisfying as the fundamental aim of nursing is to provide comfort and avoid harm. And secondly, our work has helped to raise our profile around the trust and boost our relationship with members of the health care team. Nurse practitioners and senior nurses in A/E and on the wards are keen to take on this advanced role; this would enable patients who are admitted out of hours and weekends to receive a block as close to admission as possible.

There may be challenges to overcome, which include the extensive documentation required to successfully gain approval from tiers of hospital committees, obtaining funding for equipment, and the difficulties experienced in completing the training. In spite of these hurdles it is well worth battling on, as we have proved that change can be achieved and ultimately patients benefit and the role of nursing can be advanced.

Acknowledgements

The author would like to thank the following people who have played a major role in making this service a success: Dr Barry Newman, Consultant Anaesthesia & Critical Care and clinical lead for Acute Pain Service Poole Hospital NHS Foundation Trust; Polly Cameron and Katie Horn, specialist nurses for Acute Pain Service Poole Hospital NHS Foundation Trust.

References

Arnstein, P., 2002. Optimizing perioperative pain management. *AORN Journal*, 76(5), 812–818.
Australian and New Zealand College of Anaesthetists and Faculty of Pain Medicine, 2005. *Acute Pain Management: Scientific Evidence*, 2nd edn. Available at http://www.anzca.edu.au/resources/books-and-publications/acutepain.pdf [accessed 25 August 2009].
Auory, Y., Narchi, P., Messiah, A., Litt, L., Rouvier, B., Samii, K., 1997. Serious complications related to regional anaesthesia: results of a prospective survey in France. *Anaesthesiology*, 87(3), 479–486.
Bottle, A., Aylin, P., 2006. Mortality associated with delay in operation after hip fracture: observational study. *BMJ*, 332, 947–951.
Boyd, A., Eastwood, V., Kalynych, N., McDonough, J., 2006. Clinician perceived barriers to the use of regional anaesthesia and analgesia. *Acute Pain*, 8, 23–27.
Candal-Couto, J.J., McVie, J.L., Haslam, N., Innes, A.R., Rushmer, J., 2005. Pre-operative analgesia for patients with femoral neck fractures using a modified fascia iliaca block technique. *Injury, International Journal of the Care of the Injured*, 36, 505–510.
Cohen Mansfield, J., Creedon, M., 2002. Nursing staff members' perceptions of pain indicators in persons with severe dementia. *Clinical Journal of Pain*, 18, 64–73.
Coleman, N.A., 2003 cited in Rowbotham, D.J., Macintyre, P.E., 2003. *Clinical Pain Management: Acute Pain*. Great Britain: Arnold.
Department of Health, 2001. National service framework for older people. Available at http://www.dh.gov.uk/en/publicationsandstatistics/publications/publicationspolicyandguidance/DH_4003066 [accessed 20 January 2009].
Fletcher, A., Rigby, A., Heyes, F., 2003. Three-in-one femoral nerve block as analgesia for fractured neck of femur in the emergency department: a randomized, controlled trial. *Annals of Emergency Medicine*, 41(2), 227–233.

Gullberg, B., Johnell, O., Kanis, J.A., 1997. Worldwide projections for hip fracture. *Osteoporosis International*, 7, 407–413.

Haddad, F., Williams, R., 1995. Femoral nerve block in extra capsular femoral neck fractures. *Journal of Bone and Joint Surgery (British Volume)*, 77(6), 922–923.

Harper, N., 2001. Lower limb blocks. *Current Anaesthesia and Critical Care*, 12(3), 179–185.

Hurley, K., 2004. Do femoral nerve blocks improve acute pain control in adults with isolated hip fractures? *Journal of the Canadian Association of Emergency Physicians*, 6(6), 441–443.

Institute for Innovation and Improvement, 2006. Developing quality and value. Focus on: fractured neck of femur. Available at www.institute.nhs.uk [accessed 16 March 2009].

Layzell, M.J., 2005. Improving the management of postoperative pain. *Nursing Times*, 101(26), 34–36.

Layzell, M.J., 2009. A nurse-led service for pre-operative pain management in hip fracture. *Nursing Times*, 105(3), 16–18.

Macintyre, P.E., Schug, S.A., 2007. *Acute Pain Management: A Practical Guide*, 3rd edn, China: Saunders Elsevier.

McAuliffe, L., Nay, R., O'Donnell, M., Fetherstonhaugh, D., 2009. Pain assessment in older people with dementia: literature review. *Journal of Advanced Nursing*, 65(1), 2–10.

McQuay, H., Moore, A., 1998. *An Evidence-Based Resource for Pain Relief.* New York: Oxford University Press Inc.

Morrison, R., Magaziner, J., McLaughlin, M., Orosz, G., Strauss, E., Siu, A., 2003a. Relationship between pain and opioid analgesics on the development of delirium following hip fracture. *Journal of Gerontology*, 58A(1), 76–81.

Morrison, R., Magaziner, J., McLaughlin, M., Orosz, G., Silberzweig, S., Koval, K., 2003b. The impact of post-operative pain on outcomes following hip fractures. *Pain*, 103, 303–311.

Myles, P.S., Power, I., 2007. Clinical update: postoperative analgesia. *The Lancet*, 369, 810–812.

Morrison, R., Siu, A., 2000. A comparison of pain and its treatment in advanced dementia and cognitively intact patients with hip fractures. *Journal of Pain and Symptom Management*, 19, 240–248.

Nematy, M., Hickson, M., Brynes, A., Ruxton, C., Frost, G., 2006. Vulnerable patients with a fractured neck of femur: nutritional status and support in hospital. *Journal of Human Nutrition and Dietetics*, 19, 209–218.

New Zealand Guidelines Group, 2003. Acute management and immediate rehabilitation after hip fracture amongst people aged 65 years and over. Available at http://www.nzgg.org.nz/guidelines/0006/Hip_Fracture_Prevention_Fulltext.pdf [accessed 25 August 2009].

Nursing and Midwifery Council (NMC), 2006. Advanced nursing practice update. Available at http://www.nmc-uk.org/aArticle.aspx?ArticleID=2038 [accessed 20 January 2009].

Nursing and Midwifery Council (NMC), 2008. *The Code: Standards of Conduct, Performance and Ethics for Nurses and Midwives*. London: NMC. Available at http://www.nmc-uk.org/aArticle.aspx?ArticleID=3056 [accessed 20 February 2009].

Parker, M., Johansen, A., 2006. Hip fracture. *BMJ*, 333, 27–30.

Pirmohamed, M., James, S., Meakin, S., Green, C., Scott, A., Walley, T., Farrar, K., Park, B.K., Breckenridge, A., 2004. Adverse drug reactions as cause of admission to hospital: prospective analysis of 18 820 patients. *BMJ*, 329, 15–19.

Pasero, C., McCaffrey, M., 1996. Postoperative pain management in the elderly. In Ferrell, B.R., Ferrell, B.A. (eds), *Pain in the Elderly*, pp. 45–68, Seattle WA: IASP Press.

Pasero, C., McCaffrey, M., 1997a. Overcoming obstacles to pain assessment in elders. *American Journal of Nursing*, 97, 20.

Pasero, C., McCaffrey, M., 1997b. Reluctance to order opioids in elders. *American Journal of Nursing*, 97, 21–23.

Rowbotham, D.J., Macintyre, P.E. (eds), 2003. *Clinical Pain Management: Acute Pain*. Great Britain: Arnold.

Vickers, A.P., 2007. Control of acute pain in postoperative and post-traumatic situations and the role of the acute pain service. *Anaesthesia and Intensive Care Medicine*, 9(1), 16–20.

Weiner, D.K., Hanlon, J.T., 2001. Pain in nursing home residents: management strategies. *Drugs and Ageing*, 18(1), 13–29.

Whipple, J.K., Lewis, K.S., Quebbeman, E.J., Wolff, M., Gottlieb, M.S., Medicus-Bringa, M., Hartnett, K.R., Graf, M., Ausman, R.K., 1995. Analysis of pain management in critically ill patients. *Pharmacotherapy*, 15(5), 592–599.

Williams, A., Jester, R., 2005. Delayed surgical fixation of fractured hips in older people: impact on mortality. *Journal of Advanced Nursing*, 52(1), 63–69.

Willson, H., 2000. Factors affecting the administration of analgesia to patients following repair of a fractured hip. *Journal of Advanced Nursing*, 31(5), 1145–1154.

Chapter 3
New directions in acute pain management: ketamine

Gillian Chumbley

Introduction

In November of 2002, I attended the South Thames Pain Conference and was fortunate to hear a lecture given by Professor Stephan Schug. He was discussing the concept of preventative analgesia in pain management, a medication that would reduce pain and analgesic consumption beyond the pharmacological action of the drug (McCartney *et al.* 2004). He suggested that this type of drug would be beneficial in reducing the incidence of chronic post-surgical pain.

This was a revelation for me: the prospect of administering a drug that would not only act as a painkiller, but would provide protection against developing persistent pain. The drug that could provide this level of protection was called 'ketamine'. I had heard of it, mostly in association with anaesthetics in children. Despite working in three different pain teams, over 12 years, I had only seen this drug given on one occasion. It was obvious that they were using this drug by the bucket full in Perth! I wanted to know more and was determined to visit Professor Schug at the Royal Perth Hospital, Western Australia, to see how this drug was used in practice. Almost 3 years later I made the trip and that visit changed the way that we dealt with uncontrolled pain in my own trust in West London.

Ketamine was originally synthesised in 1963 as an anaesthetic agent and was first given to American soldiers in the Vietnam War. It is useful in battlefield situations, as it produces anaesthesia without loss of respiratory drive, thereby avoiding the need for ventilation. It also preserves sympathetic reflexes, which helps to maintain blood pressure in patients who may have lost blood (Hocking *et al.* 2007).

Over 40 years later ketamine is being used in low, subanaesthetic doses for its analgesic properties, in addition to its use as an anaesthetic agent. Ketamine interacts with a number of receptors and channels and the analgesic effect is thought to be due to the antagonism of the N-methyl-D-aspartate (NMDA) receptor (Bell 2009), which is thought to be responsible for central sensitisation, the mechanism by which acute pain can become persistent (Schmid *et al.* 1999; Petrenko *et al.* 2003; Schug 2004).

In normal pain transmission, the NMDA receptor is inactive and is plugged by a magnesium ion. The pain signal enters the dorsal horn, where the primary afferent

Normal pain transmission   **Abnormal pain transmission**

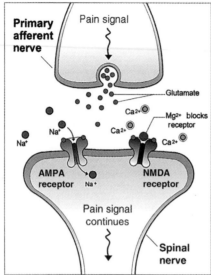
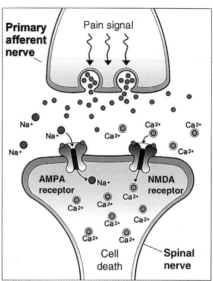

Figure 3.1 Diagram showing abnormal pain transmission when the NMDA receptor is active.

nerve synapses with the spinal nerve. For the signal to cross this gap, a chemical transmitter is required. Thus, when the pain signal enters the terminal end of the primary afferent nerve, the chemical transmitter glutamate is released. Glutamate attaches itself to an α-amino-3-hydroxy-5-methyl-4-isoxasolepropionic acid receptor on the spinal nerve and the pain message continues to the brain (see Figure 3.1).

When the dorsal horn is bombarded by pain signals and there is intense activity in the synapse, the NMDA receptor becomes active. This may occur when pain is uncontrolled after surgery, during trauma or when nerves have been injured. Activation of this receptor causes a considerable influx of calcium into the spinal nerve, which causes massive neuronal depolarisation and increases the level of excitability of this nerve (Dickenson 1997). This process is called central sensitisation and it changes the way that the nerves deal with subsequent painful stimuli (Woolf & Mannion 1999). Central sensitisation will show itself by enlarging the sensitive area of the skin that causes pain stimulation and also produces the symptoms of allodynia and hyperalgesia (Kehlet *et al.* 2006).

Allodynia occurs when a normal pleasant sensation, such as stroking the skin, causes a painful response. Patients with allodynia may dislike the sensation of having clothes or bedclothes touching the skin. Even a breeze from an open window or a fan can exacerbate pain. Hyperalgesia occurs when a minor painful stimulus, such as having a dressing or plaster removed, becomes unbearably painful. When these abnormal signs and symptoms appear, it is indicative that pain has changed from a normal noxious stimulus into a pathological process. These patients are more likely to develop persistent or chronic pain.

The neurophysiology of neuropathic pain

Clifford Woolf, a prominent researcher in this area of pain, postulates that when the NMDA receptor becomes active and there is a massive influx of calcium into the spinal nerve, this brings about the death of the nerve (Kehlet *et al.* 2006). There are many interconnecting nerves in the dorsal horn and many have an 'inhibitory' or 'switching off' function. These nerves normally have the effect of closing the pain gate and modulating the intensity of pain. If these inhibitory nerves are lost, due to activation of the NMDA receptor, the 'switching off' mechanism is absent and pain becomes persistent. Clifford Woolf suggests that pathological or neuropathic pain should be viewed as a disease process and should be actively treated to limit the long-term damage that it may cause. Medications that switch off this process are NMDA receptor antagonist, such as ketamine and, to some degree, methadone, as they block this receptor and maintain the inactive state. It is therefore the role of the professional to recognise this disease process and to ensure that the patient receives treatment.

The potential role of ketamine in chronic post-surgical pain

The concept of chronic post-surgical pain has only recently become a subject for debate. Crombie *et al.* (1998) audited why 5130 patients attended one of ten chronic pain clinics in Northern Britain. They found that 1154 (23%) patients had pain that had persisted after a surgical procedure. Of these surgical patients, 59% had pain for longer than 24 months; for 75% the pain was continuous and 76% rated their pain as moderate or severe. Research in this area is lacking, and much of the information gained has been from studies that have investigated other outcomes of surgery, rather than pain. These researchers just happened to include a question about pain. Table 3.1 shows the incidence of reported chronic post-surgical pain for some surgical procedures.

Table 3.1 Reported incidence of chronic post-surgical pain

Surgical procedure	Reported incidence (%)
Amputation	30–85
Lower limb salvage pain at 7 years	77
Thoracotomy	5–67
Mastectomy	11–57
Inguinal hernia	0–63
Cholecystectomy	3–56
Vasectomy	0–37
Dental surgery	5–37

Source: Adapted from Perkins and Kehlet (2000), Macrae (2001) and Castillo *et al.* (2006).

There are some common risk factors for developing chronic post-surgical pain (Macrae 2001) and these are:

- pre-operative pain
- uncontrolled post-operative pain
- radiotherapy or chemotherapy
- nerve damage

If persistent pain is to be avoided, then it is vital to gain control of uncontrolled post-operative pain.

So what evidence is there to support the use of ketamine in controlling pain after surgery? There have been three systematic reviews investigating this question (McCartney *et al.* 2004; Subramaniam *et al.* 2004; Bell *et al.* 2006).

McCartney *et al.* (2004) investigated whether there was a reduction in pain and analgesic consumption beyond the pharmacological action of ketamine, following a single perioperative dose. The review looked at whether ketamine was still exerting its effect five half-lives after administration. They found 24 studies where ketamine had been used in this fashion and 58% of these studies demonstrated a significant preventative effect. Most patients were receiving opioids in conjunction with ketamine and the authors suggest that one of the actions of the drug may be related to the prevention of opioid tolerance. Ketamine has proven useful when managing pain in an opioid addict because of its ability to reverse tolerance (Haller *et al.* 2002).

Subramaniam *et al.* (2004) investigated the efficacy and safety of adding low-dose ketamine as an adjuvant to perioperative opioid-based analgesia. An adjuvant is a drug that helps or assists with pain relief. Opioids were administered intravenously or epidurally; ketamine was given as a single intravenous dose, continuous infusion, with patient-controlled analgesia (PCA) or epidurally. Outcome measures included pain scores in the first 24 hours and the time that patients took to request their first dose of pain relief. Forty-five percent of trials found no benefit of adding ketamine to opioids. The authors concluded that this was because the surgical procedures were minor and the degree of post-operative pain would have been alleviated with opioids alone. In 54% studies ketamine was shown to be a useful and safe additive to opioid analgesia. The authors suggested that ketamine was most useful when used for patients having major surgical procedures that were 'difficult to manage' and where pain was not controlled with opioids. Interestingly, they found that ketamine was ineffective when it was added to opioid PCA, probably because patients received inadequate doses. Ketamine appeared to have an opioid sparing effect.

It should be noted that most commercially available preparations of ketamine contain preservatives that can be neurotoxic and should not be injected into the epidural space (Bell 2009). There are some ketamine products that are preservative free, which appear safer if they are to be administered by this route, but more research is required (Vranken *et al.* 2006; Hocking *et al.* 2007).

Bell *et al.* (2006) investigated randomised controlled trials where ketamine was administered against placebo in patients undergoing surgery. Studies were included if ketamine has been given as a single bolus dose or infusion intraoperatively, as single bolus dose or infusion post-operatively. Outcome measures included the amount of opioids used in the first 48 hours after surgery and pain intensity. Twenty-seven of the 37 trials studies found a positive effect. Ketamine reduced rescue analgesia, pain intensity and morphine requirements. Patients receiving ketamine were also found to have less nausea and vomiting, perhaps as a consequence of requiring less opioid to control pain. The authors concluded that adverse effects from ketamine were mild or absent.

One systematic review investigated whether ketamine is useful in the treatment of chronic pain (Hocking & Cousins 2003). The authors concluded that the evidence that ketamine was effective in chronic pain was moderate to weak. This was mostly due to the paucity of good quality research trials in this area. A more recent small study found ketamine to be effective in the treatment of chronic phantom limb pain (Eichenberger *et al.* 2008). Bell (2009) in a recent review concludes that information supporting the efficacy and tolerability of ketamine in the long-term treatment of chronic pain is extremely limited and further study is required. One criticism that can be levelled at many of the studies investigating the efficacy of ketamine is that the researcher did not establish whether the patient had an active NMDA receptor. If this had been established, then the results of the systematic reviews may have been more positive. It is vitally important to establish this fact in clinical practice, otherwise the drug will be administered, provide no benefit to the patient and add to the polypharmacy.

The evidence would support the use of ketamine in controlling pain after surgery and a systematic review is the highest level of evidence that can be found to indicate its effectiveness. It is therefore surprising that ketamine is not being used routinely to treat uncontrolled pain in clinical practice, in this country. Pain services have been slow to adopt it as one of the valuable weapons in our armoury to combat pain. Clinicians who are not currently using ketamine but have tried using it in the past with poor results are quick to dismiss it. It may have been their choice of patient, rather than the drug, that was at fault.

Developing the service

Having visited Perth, seen the acute pain service use ketamine in the clinical area and knowing that there was evidence to support its use in my own trust, I had to set about developing the service. My aim was to make ketamine one of the everyday drugs in our armoury of medications used to treat pain.

In 2005, my trust consisted of three separate hospital sites. I had a team of five nurses who rotated around these sites, providing acute and chronic pain relief to over 4000 inpatients per year. In addition, we ran outpatient clinics and participated in procedure lists. The service in my own hospital and in Perth differed greatly. In Perth the service was doctor-led; medical consultants conducted ward rounds 7 days a week. The ward rounds were fast moving, as the consultants had other commitments in the afternoons. There was little time for discussion with patients. The ward nurses in Perth were highly attuned to providing excellent pain relief for their patients. Very few painkillers were prescribed routinely; most were given 'as required'. The nurses were skilled and confident in administered analgesia and pain relief was at the top of their agenda, but there was little evidence for advanced nursing practice. The nurses in the pain service, though very knowledgeable, were rather in the shadow of their medical colleagues. The medical staff were rather astonished that nurses could run a pain service back in England.

In contrast, the service in my own trust was nurse-led, 5 days per week. Ward rounds were not rushed and we have time to talk, educate and discuss treatment options with our patients. The pain nurse specialists are highly qualified, most having an MSc in pain management. These nurses are working at an advanced level, advising medical teams and often anaesthetists on pain management. Unfortunately, we have a constant battle to engage ward nurses in the importance of pain relief and despite our efforts still find that 'as required' drugs are given infrequently.

I recognised that there was a need for ketamine in my own trust. Just before I had left for Perth, I had spent many hours with a young male patient who had been involved in a road traffic accident and undergone limb salvage. I had administered 50 mg of intravenous morphine to treat his pain, but this had little effect. Most patients would respond to less than 10 mg of intravenous morphine. Eventually, he was given gabapentin, a drug used for neuropathic pain. This drug has a morphine sparing effect, but it takes about 3–5 days to achieve therapeutic levels in the body. In effect, this meant waiting 3–5 days to achieve adequate pain relief. If I had had the knowledge and skills to use ketamine, this problem could have been solved in 15 minutes. Imperial College Healthcare NHS Trust is a major trauma centre and there are many surgical patients who could benefit from this advance in practice.

Ketamine should not to be used routinely for all patients. It should be restricted to patients who have active NMDA receptors. Professor Schug suggests using ketamine in patients whose pain management is difficult (Schug 2004). He gives four criteria for selecting patients:

(1) Neuropathic pain, including phantom limb pain;
(2) Patient with hyperalgesia or allodynia;
(3) Patients who respond poorly to opioids;
(4) Patients with a history of high opioid consumption preceding injury or surgery.

If the patient fulfils one or more of the above criteria, then an intravenous trial of ketamine is performed to establish whether the patient has an active NMDA receptor. Ketamine is given in 2.5 mg aliquots, at 5-minute intervals, to a maximum of 10 mg. If the patient's receptor is active, pain will reduce dramatically often from the first dose. In Perth, patients who respond are started on an intravenous infusion of ketamine. Patients receive a dose of 0.1 mg/kg/hour. Therefore, a 70 kg patient would receive 7 mg ketamine, each hour. The highly trained nursing workforce in Perth is allowed to give the patient an extra three doses of 10 mg ketamine/day. These doses provide analgesic cover for painful activities, such as dressing changes. Patients stop ketamine once the need for opioids has gone and pain requirement have greatly diminished. Patients step down to simple analgesia, such as tramadol or codeine.

Gaining stakeholder support

In order to develop the service, it was important to gain support from key stakeholders such as other members of the pain service, anaesthetists, surgeons and pharmacists. My colleagues in the pain service were hugely supportive, as they had also experienced difficulty in controlling pain of opioid-resistant patients. One of my acute pain consultant colleagues, Dr Nicola Stranix, had also heard Professor Schug's lecture in 2002 and was therefore aware of what I wanted to achieve. Her support was vital to influence her anaesthetic peer group that this was a sensible, evidence-based development. The idea of using ketamine was discussed with key anaesthetic stakeholders, such as the chief of service and the lead clinician in the intensive care unit. They were also positive about this development.

Pharmacy was another key stakeholder and helped to assess the risk of introducing this new service development in the clinical area. In terms of risk, this was an unfamiliar drug to ward nurses; they would have no knowledge of what constituted a 'normal dose' and its therapeutic effects. Others may have recognised it as an anaesthetic agent and be concerned about administering it.

One of the first steps was to develop a protocol of how we were going to manage patients who were prescribed ketamine in the trust. Unlike Perth, it was felt that our ward nurses, at that time, would not be able to cope with intravenous infusions of ketamine. Their unfamiliarity with the drug could lead to errors in calculating doses and rates when infusions were set up. Intravenous infusions of ketamine would also have required additional pumps and equipment, which would have had cost implications. The members of the pain service and pharmacy decided that ketamine should be given orally following an intravenous trial. This would require nurses to syringe 25–100 mg of ketamine from a vial, mix it with orange juice and give it to the patient (intravenous ketamine is very unpleasant to taste). This was thought to be the safest option, but was an unlicensed use of this licensed intravenous preparation. Our oral regimen started with 25 mg ketamine, three times daily. This was titrated to a maximum of 100 mg, three times daily, as required. Our oral regimen was taken from the Perth guidelines. Their pharmacy department made lozenges of ketamine that the patients sucked; our pharmacy department was unable to make lozenges, though of course I asked them. In order to reduce the dispensing risks, pharmacy suggested that a single strength of ketamine be dispensed to the ward (an ampoule of 10 mg/mL). In theatres they used much stronger solutions of 50 or 100 mg/mL and trying to measure a 25-mg dose from an ampoule of 100 mg/mL could be difficult.

Other key stakeholders were the consultant surgeons and the surgical teams responsible for the patient's treatment. The pain service acts as an advisory service to medical and surgical teams. In order to use ketamine, we needed to gain the permission of the surgical team who were responsible for the patient's care. Initially, establishing the service, we were very careful to discuss ketamine with our surgical colleagues. As you can imagine we had various comments along the lines of 'why are you using this horse tranquilliser on my patient'. It took a lot of work and effort to explain to individual surgical teams that we wanted to control pain, but were also trying to prevent persistent pain in high-risk patients. I took every opportunity that was presented to me to lecture to surgeons, anaesthetists and nurses on the subject of chronic post-surgical pain. My impression was that many professionals were oblivious to the fact that pain could persist after surgery.

Protocols, guidelines and policies

Any nurse working in the field of pain management strives to prevent patients going through unnecessary discomfort. You are enthusiastic to embrace new evidence-based interventions and can find the slow pace of change frustrating, especially when others are hesitant or disinclined to alter their practice. There is a tendency to rush ahead, without putting all of the necessary apparatus in place. You know that you have the key to the problem and do not want to get hindered by paperwork. We certainly had a verbal protocol in place, but it took us some time to write a formal guideline. This was obviously not a problem for the team, as we knew what we were doing in these first few patients, but it would have been logical to have a written guideline and information for the staff and patients before we started. We had research articles, but not everyone has the inclination or ability to read them. Formulating easily understood information leaflets could have helped with communication. Nowadays we have guidelines which are available on our hospital intranet. In addition to this, it would have been easier if we had set up the mechanisms for audit, prior to starting the service. When I finally came to audit our practice, I had to retrieve the patients' notes from the archives, which was a very time-consuming activity.

It was important to educate the nursing staff on this new intervention. Initially we did not know how many patients would require ketamine, whether this would become an established practice and therefore felt awkward in teaching nurses formally, on our pain study day, about the drug they may never use. We usually insist that at least 75% of nurses working on surgical wards attend this study day. At first, most of the patients were situated on the orthopaedic wards and initially teaching took place at the bedside, educating individual nurses. Once the practice had become more established, we incorporated the management of patients having ketamine into our formal pain study day.

One other consideration that had to be taken into account when developing this new practice was our trust's sedation policy. The policy states that 'ketamine can only be given by or in the presence of an anaesthetist'. So having identified a patient that fitted the criteria for a ketamine trial, the pain service had to call the anaesthetist to administer it. Although this was not ideal and there would be a delay waiting for the anaesthetist, this policy was going to be difficult to change. Policy changes would have involved getting agreement from several committees, which only met monthly and there would have been a wait to get this item on an agenda. Interestingly, some committees would only accept changes presented by medical consultants, rather than nurses. In practice, I could prescribe this drug, but not administer it.

We were going to have to work with the restrictions of the sedation policy. But there were benefits to this restriction, as we would be educating consultant and junior anaesthetists how to use ketamine in difficult pain patients. Having seen the benefits of this drug in action, they may be more inclined to use this therapy again, perhaps on patients they were called to see out of hours.

Challenges in implementing a new service or area of practice development

There were certainly many challenges that the service had to face. The first one was the attitude of clinicians to this particular drug. It appeared that everyone had an opinion about ketamine, which was not based on scientific evidence. I do not think that I can remember a drug that so many people felt negatively about. It is difficult to decipher why this should be. Was it because it can cause patients to dissociate? Was it due to this drug being used recreationally for veterinary medicine or because we were using anaesthetic agents in the ward environment? It may have been due to one or a combination of these reasons, but mostly the negativity stemmed from ignorance about the actions of this drug. More of a case that a little knowledge is a dangerous thing! There were times when I wished that we could have called it something else, just to take away the negative connotations.

Clinicians, especially surgeons, could not understand why we were giving an anaesthetic agent to their patients. They had no concept of what would constitute an anaesthetic or analgesic dose; they just reacted to the name. On many occasions we would explain our rationale to the senior registrar, who in the absence of the consultant would agree to use ketamine, only to find it had been stopped on the consultant's weekly ward round. I am astonished that surgeons have no perception that the operations they perform can cause pain, either acute or chronic. As pain clinicians we are partly to blame; articles about chronic post-surgical pain are rarely published in surgical journals and therefore this subject is off the surgeon's radar. For example, not one of the articles that I have referenced for this chapter has been published in a specific surgical journal.

In the struggle to win over the surgeons there were many situations like these, but eventually they saw the benefit of using ketamine, and now 3 years later we rarely have a problem. Many of the difficulties arose from a lack of knowledge and poor communication. In hindsight, it would have been preferable to try to find a forum to discuss the use of this drug with the surgical consultants. But there are always huge difficulties in getting this group of clinicians together at the same time. On the whole, there were few problems with the junior doctors, who were just grateful that we had managed to sort out their most difficult patient and were on hand to see the dramatic results.

Ketamine is associated with veterinary medicine. Ironically the very first patient that we treated with ketamine was a jockey, so he was very familiar with the drug. But this was the reason why doctors would refer to it being a 'horse tranquilliser'. Many of the younger patients knew that this drug was used for recreational use.

Most clinicians were concerned about the adverse effects of ketamine. When it is given in anaesthetic doses, it can produce hallucinations, agitation, nightmares, dizziness and nausea (Bell 2009). It is a dissociative anaesthetic and therefore patients tend to lose their grip on reality. When ketamine is first given as an anaesthetic it has a sympathomimetic effect and will raise the patient's blood pressure and pulse rate. But in subanaesthetic doses, patient rarely experience side effects (Schmid *et al.* 1999; Schug 2004; Himmelseher & Durieux 2005; Bell *et al.* 2006; Hocking *et al.* 2007). In practice, we did monitor patients when we were loading them, but had no problems with sympathomimetic effects.

Cases of tolerance to ketamine have been reported in children when the drug has been used repeatedly in anaesthetic doses (Tobias 2000). There is minimal evidence to show that cessation of subanaesthetic doses of ketamine produces withdrawal syndrome in adults. But one case report describes generalised hyperalgesia and allodynia following abrupt cessation of a subcutaneous infusion of ketamine in a cancer patient (Mitchell 1999). There have been reported difficulties in stopping this drug in patients using ketamine recreationally, who have taken doses of up to 4 g/day. This was due to psychological dependence rather than any physical withdrawal (Lim 2003). One other author reported insomnia as the only obvious physical sign of withdrawal during dependence detoxification (Pal *et al.* 2002).

With any new intervention, you endeavour to assess and minimise the risks to the patient. In our initial assessment we chose not to administer ketamine intravenously, as we felt that our staff were unfamiliar with it and mistakes in drawing up intravenous solutions could result in patients receiving anaesthetic doses of the drug. We discussed our proposals with pharmacy and ensured that one strength of ketamine was dispensed to the ward. Unfortunately, on one occasion a higher strength ampoule was dispensed: the ward nurses did not read the label and the patient received ten times the stated oral dose. At this dose the patient did experience hallucinations and dissociation and understandably refused to take the drug again. Midazolam can be given to correct this adverse effect (Schug 2004; Hocking *et al.* 2007).

As a result of this clinical incident, an oral suspension of ketamine was obtained to prevent further errors in its administration. The suspension has proven to be very useful, easier to administer and has been safer to use. Our colleagues in the pharmacy department were highly supportive of what we wanted to achieve with ketamine and following this incident, caused by chain of human errors, never suggested that we should withdraw the service. Their reaction was a measured response to strive to make administration even safer.

This unwanted clinical incident did, however, confirm the safety of this drug. If a nurse had administered ten times the prescribed dose of other analgesic drugs, the outcomes would have been very different.

Evaluation of using ketamine for pain relief

Hindsight is a great asset, but it is a shame that we cannot possess this knowledge in advance. In my rush to treat difficult patients, I failed to set up a system to audit the outcomes of using ketamine in practice. This lapse first became apparent when I was asked to talk to the orthopaedic surgeons about pain management. I wanted to take this opportunity to educate the consultants about the benefits of using ketamine, but had no data to present. Similarly, this lack of data became evident when I was asked to talk at an international pain meeting about the introduction of ketamine to the inpatient service. I could not lecture unless I had original data about the effectiveness. There was no choice but to conduct a retrospective audit. This required hours of sifting through pain audit sheets to identify the patients who had used it. The medical notes had to be retrieved from filing and I spent four weekends rummaging through notes to extract the required data. This would have been avoided with the correct preparation.

Despite the personal effort involved, it was a very worthwhile exercise because it provided the evidence to show that ketamine had made a difference and improved the pain relief for our patients. In the process I created an audit sheet, so data collection would be ongoing. The types of data we collect are given below:

- Sample information: gender, age, ward, surgical specialty;
- Diagnosis and/or type of surgery performed;
- Reason for starting ketamine (from four criteria given above);
- Analgesic regimen prior to starting ketamine;
- Pain scores pre- and post-ketamine trial;
- Loading dose given;
- Starting dose of ketamine;
- Titrations of ketamine dose;
- Total number of days taking ketamine;
- Other medications: especially pain medications and adjuvants.

Prior to the introduction of ketamine, difficult patients who were unresponsive to opioids were prescribed an anticonvulsant drug called gabapentin. This is given to treat neuropathic pain, but gabapentin also has a morphine sparing effect. Many patients cannot tolerate the side effects of this drug, which include weight gain, sedation and difficulty with cognition. Patients may need to take this drug for many months, which can also reduce concordance. By auditing the use of ketamine, I wanted to establish how many patients had benefited from the protective aspects of ketamine and avoided having to be treated with gabapentin. There would obviously be monetary savings, as it costs approximately £30–90 per month to treat a patient with gabapentin, depending on the dose. But this would be offset by the cost of ketamine suspension, which depending on the dose could cost between £10 and £30 per day.

A sample of 45 patients who had been prescribed ketamine was audited. The mean age of the sample was 45 years (range 20–74 years). Ketamine appears to be well tolerated by all patients regardless of age. The majority were young men who had been involved in road traffic accidents and had undergone limb salvage or amputation. The average time spent on ketamine was 21 days, but this mean was heavily skewed by one patient who required the drug for 103 days. This patient was an elderly lady who had an infected knee replacement. She had multiple operations, which included removal of the prosthesis and eventually a high above knee amputation. Despite many surgical procedures, ketamine appeared to protect her from developing phantom pain. We use normal doses in patients with renal impairment. The only patients we tend to exclude are patients with schizophrenia, as the dissociative effects can mimic some of these symptoms.

Table 3.2   Patients' pain scores before and after receiving an intravenous trial of ketamine

Pain score	Number and percentage of patients	
	Pre-ketamine ($n = 43$)	Post-ketamine ($n = 39$)
None	0	3 (8)
Mild	0	19 (49)
Moderate	2 (5)	14 (36)
Severe	21 (49)	1 (3)
Unbearable	20 (46)	2 (5)

Most patients who were prescribed ketamine had been using PCA, when they were found to have uncontrolled post-operative pain. The most common selection criterion was acute neuropathic pain. Patient's pain was scored before and after the intravenous trial of ketamine and these results are presented in Table 3.2.

There was a statistically significant difference in pain scores pre- and post-ketamine trial. Three patients did not respond and were left with severe or unbearable pain. These patients were deemed not to have an active NMDA receptor and other methods of pain relief were sought. For the majority, ketamine reduced their pain scores from severe or unbearable to mild.

The audit established that most patients were changed from a dose of 25 mg, three times daily to a four times daily dosing regimen. The oral regimen was taken from the Perth guidelines, where they prescribed lozenges three times daily. Further work by their department has established that the bioavailability of oral ketamine is lower than the bioavailability for sublingual ketamine. This difference is the likely reason why patients have required a different dosing regimen. As a result of the audit, we now start all patients on a four times per day dosing regimen.

Thirty-five percent patients in the audit were taking medications for neuropathic pain, such as gabapentin or amitriptyline, prior to starting ketamine. By the time ketamine was discontinued this number had risen to 51%. As mentioned previously, before the introduction of ketamine, all patients would have been commenced on these types of drugs. It would therefore appear that we had prevented 49% patient from having to take these medications.

Justifying the advanced nursing contribution

There is still some debate as to what constitutes advanced nursing practice, though many would agree that it comprises the sub-roles of educator, researcher and consultant (Por 2008). In the last decade there has been a melding of nursing and medical roles within pain services. What was seen as the domain of the anaesthetist or physician has been cultivated and developed by nurses who are highly trained, often to a master or doctorate level, as I have been. Nurses have the advantage of working within the pain service full time and can devote more hours to its expansion. The role of the consultant nurse has allowed services to advance a stage further by treating their own clinical caseload and having designated time for education and research. That is not to say that nurses should work in isolation; the best developments occur when there is a multidisciplinary approach.

Therefore, did the introduction of ketamine for pain management constitute advanced nursing practice? In order to change practice in the trust, I had to use all the aforementioned sub-roles. I also question whether practice would have changed if I had not been the driver. I suspect that the odd dose of ketamine may have been used when nothing else worked. The approach to its utilisation would not have been well researched; criteria and protocols would not have been established and audit not performed. It would not have become a standard drug in our armoury of pain relief. This change was driven by nurses, led by the nurse consultant and the success of its adoption was due to the chipping away of old attitudes and the belief that we could provide a better service for patients.

In fairness to my anaesthetic colleagues, they may not have been aware of the gap in pain provision, as the management of post-surgical pain has become the domain of the nurse-led pain service. But as mentioned previously, I had only seen this drug used once to treat pain in the past 14 years. Ketamine was not considered an effective drug in the management of pain.

To adopt a new method of working into routine practice, it takes an individual who is passionate about the benefits, who has collated the scientific evidence, has recognised a gap in the management of patients and who can identify how the change can be incorporated into current practice. This is made easier if you are known and respected by the organisation. This trust is built up over time as your colleagues begin to see the positive changes that have been brought about by the application of your knowledge and skills. Although the sub-roles of educator, researcher and consultant are the basic requirements to move practice forward, it is essential to be recognised as an experienced expert in your field.

An advanced practitioner has to have a working knowledge of the scientific evidence and be comfortable conversing with colleagues, from a range of professions, at this level. For advanced nursing practice to be taken seriously, we have to use the correct language. Higher educational degrees give nurses the confidence, knowledge and skills to recognise, disseminate and utilise robust research.

A large part of my role over the past 3 years in establishing the use of ketamine has been one of educator and consultant. There has been a role reversal; anaesthetic colleagues contact me for advice, rather than the traditional roles of nurses seeking advice from anaesthetists. Curiosity about ketamine has not just emanated from clinicians within my own trust; colleagues in other parts of the country and Ireland have been interested in our work.

Advanced nursing practice requires nurses to be innovative and to develop services that will improve patient care. It requires nurses to provide leadership, to develop expertise and autonomy. We have to recognise the need to audit and critically assess progress to check that change is truly benefiting patients.

Conclusions

Over the last 3 years I have sought to change our pain service from one that not only deals with the immediate problem of pain relief for our patients, but is also concerned with the prevention of chronic pain. This has required patience, enthusiasm and motivation to change the practice of not only my immediate pain colleagues, but also the attitudes of surgical teams. After 3 years I can proudly claim that ketamine is a drug that is used routinely in the trust; it is an established practice and we continue to educate junior anaesthetists to the advantages of using it in difficult patients. The eureka moment came when I discovered our junior anaesthetists initiating this treatment out of hours, when the pain service was off duty. The primary role of any pain service should be one of education; the service must function in our absence.

In the process of change you always learn from your mistakes. In hindsight we could have improved communication with our surgical colleagues, but there is much to be said for a slow chipping away of attitudes and for consultants gaining confidence in our ability to improve pain relief for their patients. You earn respect and trust through your ability to control pain in difficult situations, with each individual patient.

In any future projects I would automatically set up a system of audit from the beginning. It is crucial to be able to ascertain the advantages or disadvantages of changing practice and to provide evidence to convince your colleagues of the benefits.

Assessing and preventing risks is mandatory, but however careful you are, there are always clinical incidents that you have not foreseen. It would have been preferable to have sourced oral ketamine suspension prior to setting up the service. It was only following the error that we investigated whether a supplier could be found. Having never seen this product before, it was not something that even occurred to me. In fact, it was the pharmacy department who was responsible for this breakthrough. Currently an intranasal version of ketamine is going through Phase 3 trials in Europe and the USA for its use in trauma and post-operative patients. In the future we could be using this method of administration, which would certainly help patients who are nil by mouth.

In my clinical area I can prescribe ketamine for patients, but cannot actually administer it unless I have an anaesthetist present, because of the stipulations of our local sedation policy. I have agreement from the anaesthetic consultants that clinical nurse specialists in the pain service should be able to administer analgesic doses of ketamine, but as with every other organisation there are several committees to go through before policies can be changed. I am in two minds about changing this policy. It has meant a delay in treating patients, as we have had to find an anaesthetist. In practice this only holds back treatment by minutes, but any delay for a patient is intolerable. On the plus side, this restriction has allowed us to educate the junior anaesthetists, which is essential. Junior anaesthetists will change hospitals and hopefully take these skills with them. When the policy does change, we will have to think of innovative ways to train our anaesthetic colleagues.

With further education, publications and lectures, I am hopeful that we can influence other pain services to adopt this advanced nursing practice. In doing so, we will save patients from having to live with chronic pain.

References

Bell, R.F., 2009. Ketamine for chronic non-cancer pain. *Pain*, 141, 210–214.

Bell, R.F., Dahl J.B., Moore R.A., Kalso E., 2006. Perioperative ketamine for acute postoperative pain. *Cochrane Database Systematic Review* (1): CD004603.

Castillo, R.C., MacKenzie, E.J., Wegener, S.T., Bosse, M.J., 2006. Prevalence of chronic pain seven years following limb threatening lower extremity trauma. *Pain*, 124(3), 321–329.

Crombie, I.K., Davies, H.T., Macrae, W.A., 1998. Cut and thrust: antecedent srgery and trauma among patients attending a chronic pain clinic. *Pain*, 76(1–2), 167–171.

Dickenson, A.H., 1997. NMDA receptor antagonists: interactions with opioids. *Acta Anaesthesiologica Scandinavica*, 41(1 Pt 2), 112–115.

Eichenberger, U., Neff, F., Sveticic, G., Bjorgo, S., Petersen-Felix, S., Arendt-Nielsen, L., Curatolo, M., 2008. Chronic phantom limb pain: the effects of calcitonin, ketamine, and their combination on pain and sensory thresholds. *Anesthesia and Analgesia*, 106(4), 1265–1273.

Haller, G., Waeber, J.L., Infante, N.K., Clergue, F., 2002. Ketamine combined with morphine for the management of pain in an opioid addict. *Anesthesiology*, 96(5), 1265–1266.

Himmelseher, S., Durieux, M.E., 2005. Ketamine for perioperative pain management. *Anesthesiology*, 102(1), 211–220.

Hocking, G., Cousins, M.J., 2003. Ketamine in chronic pain management: an evidence-based review. *Anesthesia and Analgesia*, 97(6), 1730–1739.

Hocking, G., Visser, E.J., Schug, S.A., Cousins, M.J., 2007. Ketamine: does life begin at 40? *Pain: Clinical Updates*, XV(3), 1–6.

Kehlet, H., Jensen, T.S., Woolf, C.J., 2006. Persistent post surgical pain: risk factors and prevention. *Lancet*, 367(9522), 1618–1625.

Lim, D.K., 2003. Ketamine associated psychedelic effects and dependence. *Singapore Medical Journal*, 44(1), 31–34.

Macrae, W.A., 2001. Chronic pain after surgery. *British Journal of Anaesthesia*, 87(1), 88–98.

McCartney, C.J., Sinha, A., Katz, J., 2004. A qualitative systematic review of the role of N-methyl-D-aspartate receptor antagonists in preventive analgesia. *Anesthesia and Analgesia*, 98(5), 1385–1400.

Mitchell, A.C., 1999. Generalized hyperalgesia and allodynia following abrupt cessation of subcutaneous ketamine infusion. *Palliative Medicine*, 13(5), 427–428.

Pal, H.R., Berry, N., Kumar, R., Ray, R., 2002. Ketamine dependence. *Anaesthesia and Intensive Care*, 30(3), 382–384.

Perkins, F.M., Kehlet, H., 2000. Chronic pain as an outcome of surgery. A review of predictive factors. *Anesthesiology*, 93(4), 1123–1133.

Petrenko, A.B., Yamakura, T., Baba, H., Shimoji, K., 2003. The role of N-methyl-D-aspartate (NMDA) receptors in pain: a review. *Anesthesia and Analgesia*, 97(4), 1108–1116.

Por, J., 2008. A critical engagement with the concept of advancing nursing practice. *Journal of Nursing Management*, 16(1), 84–90.

Schmid, R.L., Sandler, A.N., Katz, J., 1999. Use and efficacy of low-dose ketamine in the management of acute postoperative pain: a review of current techniques and outcomes. *Pain*, 82(2), 111–125.

Schug, S.A., 2004. New uses for an old drug: the role of ketamine in post-operative pain management. *ASEAN Journal of Anaesthesiology*, 5(1), 39–42.

Subramaniam, K., Subramaniam, B., Steinbrook, R.A., 2004. Ketamine as adjuvant analgesic to opioids: a quantitative and qualitative systematic review. *Anesthesia and Analgesia*, 99(2), 482–495.

Tobias, J.D., 2000. Tolerance, withdrawal, and physical dependency after long-term sedation and analgesia of children in the pediatric intensive care unit. *Critical Care Medicine*, 28(6), 2122–2213.

Vranken, J.H., Troost, D., de Haan, P., Pennings, F.A, Van Der Vegt, M.H., Dijkgraaf, M.G., Hollmann, M.W., 2006. Severe toxic damage to the rabbit spinal cord after intrathecal administration of preservative-free S (+)-ketamine. *Anesthesiology*, 105(4), 813–818.

Woolf, C.J., Mannion, R.J., 1999. Neuropathic pain: aetiology, symptoms, mechanisms, and management. *Lancet*, 353(9168), 1959–1964.

Chapter 4
Developing a nurse-led clinic for the treatment of neuropathic pain

Eileen Mann

Introduction

Neuropathic pain is an extremely challenging condition to treat. It is often an undiagnosed feature of chronic pain and because of the type of pain experienced, it is generally resistant to treatment with commonly prescribed analgesics (Orza *et al.* 2000). Data continue to suggest that the clinical management of neuropathic pain is inadequate and ineffective. Patients with neuropathic pain visit their doctor frequently, experience poor health-related quality of life and consume a high level of health care resources (Taylor 2006). A large proportion of patients continue to report substantial pain despite receiving treatment, and for many patients their employment status will be negatively affected (McDermott *et al.* 2006). Failure to recognise, assess and manage chronic neuropathic pain in a logical, multimodal and evidence-based fashion can have a devastating impact on patients and their families. So severe can the impact of neuropathic pain become that suicidal thoughts and intentions are not uncommon (Fishbain 1999).

Definitions and causes of neuropathic pain

Neuropathic pain can be described as pain related to abnormal processing within the nervous system. The International Association for the Study of Pain defines it as 'pain initiated or caused by a primary lesion or dysfunction of the nervous system' (Merskey & Bogduk 1994) and more recently it has been referred to as a consequence of injury or disease affecting the peripheral and/or central nervous systems associated with various sensory and/or motor phenomena (Backonja 2003). Pain continues beyond the normal period of tissue healing and its relentless persistence is associated with serious comorbidity and major disability (Cavenagh *et al.* 2006; Gustorff *et al.* 2008). We now know nerve damage can change the biochemistry and anatomic circuitry, not only of primary sensory afferents but also of spinal and even brain neurons. This reorganisation associated with neuropathic pain opens up pharmacological and non-pharmacological strategies that would not be effective for the treatment of nociceptive pain. Unfortunately, evidence suggests that health care professionals continue to treat neuropathic pain as they would treat nociceptive pain and this may contribute to the failure of many patients to obtain improved pain control.

There are numerous causes of neuropathic pain. For instance, nerve injury can result from infection, trauma, metabolic disorder, chemotherapy, surgery, radiation, neurotoxins, nerve compression and tumour infiltration. Common conditions that can lead to painful damage to peripheral nerves include diabetic neuropathy and post-herpetic neuralgia, whilst conditions such as post-stroke pain and spinal cord damage are associated with disruption to part of the central nervous system.

Prevalence of neuropathic pain

Neuropathic pain is common with some estimates, suggesting approximately 1.3% of the US population may suffer from neuropathic pain syndromes (Bennett 1997). More recent estimates within the UK population put the incidence of neuropathic pain at approximately 1.5% (Taylor 2006) whilst pain with a neuropathic component is estimated to be as high as 8% (Torrance *et al.* 2005). Despite this high incidence, access to effective treatment regimes is limited. A Danish study found that only 7% of patients with spinal cord injury received drugs and considered to be effective (Finnerup *et al.* 2001). In the USA an earlier study found that only 12% of neuropathic pain patients were treated with a potentially effective drug prescribed at an appropriate dose (Richeimer *et al.* 1997) and from a later European study the situation had not substantially improved (Hans *et al.* 2007).

Alarmingly many general practitioners (GPs) as well as non-pain specialists such as diabetologists or neurologists fail to diagnose or manage neuropathic pain (Harden & Cohen 2003). Misdiagnosis or a lack of understanding of pain mechanisms by non-specialists is recognised to be a problem throughout the world (Harden & Cohen 2003). In one Japanese study involving 6472 patients with diabetes, 85% were found to have neurological symptoms, yet only half of these patients were identified as having diabetic neuropathy (Kawena *et al.* 2001). Despite the growing number of chronic pain clinics, only a small proportion of patients with chronic neuropathic pain are referred to a pain specialist and of those over three quarters have had the condition for more than 1 year before obtaining a specialist referral (Davies *et al.* 1994).

A study by McDermott *et al.* (2006) indicated some improved medication regimes; however, the indications were that the medications selected did not reduce patient visits to their doctors or lead to improved outcomes. It is generally considered that the earlier treatment for neuropathic pain is initiated the more likelihood there is of reducing symptoms. Delays, ineffective medications or failure to address the psychosocial implications of pain may add to the risks of long-term disability, chronicity and poor quality of life.

A high proportion of patients with neuropathic pain will go on to develop comorbid conditions such as depression, anxiety and insomnia. Indeed, some studies report a prevalence rate for depression in chronic pain patients as high as 100% (Fishbain 1999). As many patients with neuropathic pain will report symptoms that are worse at night, it does not come as a surprise that between 60 and 70% will suffer sleep disturbance

(Zelman *et al.* 2006; Gustorff *et al.* 2008). This in turn can have a negative impact on pain perception, coping strategies, quality of life and work status. Alarmingly, recent evidence suggests that sleep disorders may contribute to the development of pathophysiological changes associated with the development of type 2 diabetes (Morritt Taub & Redeker 2008). We knew that neuropathic pain contributed to sleep deprivation, but only recently that sleep deprivation may contribute to neuropathic pain.

A proposal and rationale for a nurse-led clinic for sufferers of neuropathic pain

The purpose of this chapter is to discuss a proposal for the introduction of a nurse-led clinic to help treat neuropathic pain based ideally in primary care. It will discuss why a service such as this is needed and explore further the factors that contribute to the current inadequate management of neuropathic pain. It will also explore how a service can be developed and who the key stakeholders may be. Although in this instance the proposal suggested is nurse-led, the reality is that the template for such a clinic could be relevant to any clinician wishing to pursue such a development. The use of audit and evaluation will be described, as well as the challenges that can be anticipated. Acknowledging the challenges and overcoming barriers will be a key feature. Although the development of any non-medical practitioner-led clinic may be controversial, the need to challenge current strategies and the status quo is vital and timely with government initiatives such as 'Our health, our care, our say' (Department of Health [DH] 2006).

What we all are going to face in the future is an increasing incidence of neuropathic pain (Dworkin 2002). As populations age, both non-malignant and malignant diseases will increase. Obesity and the rise of metabolic disorders appear to be inevitable within industrialised nations. In addition, increasing numbers of people are now living with chronic conditions associated with the development of neuropathic pain such as cancer, HIV/AIDS and multiple sclerosis that may previously have proved fatal at a much earlier age. The burdens on GPs are great and their diagnostic skills are key; however, advanced practice nurses are well placed to implement rational, evidence-based care pathways to help manage complex and chronically painful conditions such as neuropathic pain.

Despite recent advances in our knowledge of the conditions that may lead to neuropathic pain, only a limited number of effective treatments are available with a wide variability in patient response. Our inability to establish a precise pain generator makes managing this condition far more complex than the treatment of much of the pain encountered in primary care. A study in 2006 by McDermott *et al.* indicated that 76% of patients with neuropathic pain had visited their GP at least once in the past month, despite this 54% of patients with neuropathic pain rated their pain as moderate, with 25% reporting severe pain. Because of pain and resulting comorbidities, patients reported that their employment status was affected, with those in employment missing an average of 5.5 workdays a month. In the USA a study conducted over 3 months with patients suffering from painful diabetic neuropathy indicated nearly 60% of patients had two health professional consults, 59% reported decreased home productivity, 85.5% reported activity limitations and 64.4% of patients who worked reported missing work or decreased work productivity due to their neuropathic pain. These results confirm the high burden on patients, their families, employers and society in general despite the current input of health care resources. The results also suggest sub-optimal pain management and low levels of satisfaction with treatments (Gore *et al.* 2006). Attempts to improve the management of neuropathic pain appear to be hampered by inadequate diagnosis, a lack of appreciation of the mechanisms involved, insufficient management of comorbidity, incorrect understanding or selection of treatment options and the use of inappropriate outcomes measures (Harden & Cohen 2003).

Many nurses as well as other health care professionals have developed a keen interest in pain management. This is probably in some part due to the frustration of being with patients who remain in inadequately treated pain and feeling powerless to provide more effective therapies. Nurses may feel that their initial education did not prepare them adequately to deal with patients suffering from complex pain. However, nurses spend more time with patients in pain than any other health care professional, and certainly in secondary care, they cannot withdraw when pain relief is poor. In the past decade or so, significant numbers of nurses have undertaken postgraduate and post-registration higher education in pain management, and in some cases to master's and even to doctorate level. With the addition of prescribing rights for clinicians who have undergone specific training, developing clinics run by nurses for the management of established neuropathic pain would seem to be a logical and effective way of utilising their skills and specialist knowledge more effectively.

Patients with neuropathic pain will rarely respond first time to just one or two treatment regimes. Their care can be time-consuming and challenging, requiring the trail of a wide range of drugs and therapies at varying dosages and with varying degrees of success before the most effective treatment regime can be established. This is combined with the fact that only about 30% of patients will respond to any of the so far established medications. These somewhat disappointing results mean an achievable treatment goal using pharmacological strategies alone may realistically only be a 20–30% reduction in their pain. Any effective strategies must therefore involve a potentially lengthy and detailed assessment process involving medication and non-pharmacological treatment trials. Perhaps more important, though, is having the time to listen to the problems of sufferers, providing the opportunity to educate patients and their families about the condition and the various treatment options available, empowering patients to take control of their lives and enhancing self-help coping strategies. When pain cannot be entirely relieved, we often overlook patients' own resources to cope, to come to terms with their pain and improve their quality of life. With improved knowledge of their condition and by becoming a key part of a team, it is possible to achieve improved and tangible outcomes for these patients. Many of the patients I encountered were just so relieved to know that their pain was 'real' and not 'all in the mind'. Having the diagnosis of neuropathic pain and an explanation of what this was seemed to lift a huge burden off many patients. As one patient said, '[I]t makes such a difference knowing your enemy'.

Developing the service

The following section will reflect my development of such a nurse-led service. It was established in 2004 within the Diabetic Department of a District General Hospital. Although many people were subsequently involved, the initial proposal developed following discussion with physicians in acute medicine and it was initially designed to manage the pain of patients suffering from painful diabetic neuropathy. In reality, as you would probably expect, the clinic uncovered a wide range of pain, particularly musculoskeletal and visceral pain in this patient group, but given the limitations of a single chapter, I shall concentrate on the rationale, structure and process for the management of just neuropathic pain.

My interest was developed from seeing patients in secondary care, who had not been admitted with an obvious cause of their pain such as trauma or an acutely painful medical condition. So many of these patients had never had the source or generator of their pain investigated, assessed or established where that was possible, even when the risk of developing neuropathic pain was high, such as following an attack of shingles. To them, and indeed some of their clinicians, pain was just pain and a lack of response to prescribed analgesia was unfortunate and something they would have to learn to live with. Given the explosion of interest and research into neuropathic pain over the past 10 years, this seemed to be an area where pain relief and outcomes could be improved. In hindsight, I was fairly naive in thinking it would be reasonably straightforward to develop such a service.

Rationale for management

At the time my rationale looked fairly clear. I hoped to increase liaison between primary and secondary care. I wanted to improve the diagnosis and assessment of neuropathic pain, enhance patients' coping strategies, improve pain control and relieve side effects using a range of pharmacological and non-pharmacological therapies. These would be based on the latest available evidence and, where possible, follow an agreed algorithm or care pathway. With the development of a wide range of validated assessment tools, I intended to undertake a comprehensive assessment of pain intensity, confirm the presence of neuropathic pain as well as the impact of pain on patients' functional status and daily activities. Other issues including sleep disturbance and fatigue would be assessed, as well as psychosocial factors such as depression, anxiety, fear avoidance and withdrawal from previously pleasurable pursuits. I intended the clinic to provide an opportunity for erroneous beliefs and misconceptions to be explored, discussed and hopefully addressed. In fact, education proved to be a key intervention.

Evaluation of pharmacological strategies including efficacy, duration of action and side effects would follow an agreed algorithm. I also intended to trial non-pharmacological strategies deemed appropriate, such as behaviour change skills. Behaviour change skills are seen as important in influencing health status. These are a combination of psychological approaches, which can be applied in traditional clinical settings and are evidence-based. These are 'motivational approaches' (adapted from motivational interviewing) and 'cognitive behavioural approaches' (adapted from cognitive–behavioural therapy) (Turk & Gatchel 2002).

The clinic would also offer an opportunity to provide patients with as much information as possible. This would include providing booklets such as 'Opioid medicines for persistent pain: information for patients' produced by the British Pain Society (2004a) for any patients whose treatment included a trial of strong opioids. Additional information sheets were developed to accompany any other pharmacological strategies that were commenced. I also obtained a large quantity of booklets for patients produced by the Neuropathy Trust, which were very informative and provided patients with the opportunity to subscribe to this organisation should they wish. Where possible, involvement with reputable charitable organisations associated with pain management and self-help groups such as the expert patient programme was encouraged.

A care plan and patient-held diary that informs the patient and their GP of their treatment with further options to be considered was introduced. Treatment options were listed according to strength of supporting evidence. (Duplicate data were included in patient's notes and could easily be transferred to an electronic patient record.) The diary was designed to improve evaluation of strategies, enhance communication and avoid the reuse of medications already deemed to have failed or which had contributed to unacceptable side effects in the past. Agreed goals could be made explicit to help patients achieve the best possible functional status and quality of life. This document would help to assure patients that their pain was being taken seriously, that there was a logical pathway to their care and that all relevant health care professionals had access to this information. In doing this, it was hoped to avoid some of the iatrogenic damage that can occur when patients are prescribed ineffective or inappropriate medication, patients fail to have access to the latest evidence-based treatment, or appropriate treatment is delayed until pain has become intractable.

Identifying stakeholders

In order to get anything like this up and running, identifying key stakeholders was vital. I needed powerful initial supporters such as a senior medical clinician and the director of nursing. I was based at the time in secondary care, and although I felt a neuropathic pain clinic should be located in primary care, in order to trial the system and get something started it was initially agreed that I could undertake a weekly clinic within the Diabetic Department seeing patients on an outpatient basis as a pilot project. I needed to develop a business plan to present to the local Primary Care Trusts and Secondary Care Trust Board (see Appendix 1 for a copy of the original business plan). Contacting people in the voluntary sector such as the Neuropathy Trust was helpful, and representatives of patient groups were also contacted to gain their views. Particularly, individuals from the expert patient group were invaluable and very supportive.

I discussed the proposal with senior clinicians, particularly the physicians to whom patients may be referred with medical conditions more likely to result in neuropathic pain such as neurologists, consultants for diabetes, geriatricians and palliative care specialists. Although initially the service was going to be established for patients with painful diabetic neuropathy, if it was intended to extend to other neuropathic pain in the future, it would be useful to include physicians who specialise in chronic diseases with a neuropathic component such as multiple sclerosis, Parkinson's disease and AIDS. I contacted the consultants involved in the running of the pain clinic, as the intention was ultimately to ensure they only received referrals for patients for whom all treatments based on an agreed algorithm had failed. They were available for telephone advice and were very supportive as it was hoped in time initiating therapy; in primary care it could impact on their waiting times.

I then wrote an open letter to all the local GPs, informing them of the proposal to develop the service and requesting comment from primary care (see Appendix 2). I followed this up with an article in the local GP newsletter along similar lines. Other key stakeholders included nursing staff, particularly specialist diabetic practitioners, podiatrists, relevant administration staff, receptionists and clerical staff in the diabetic centre responsible for booking the outpatient clinics and obtaining notes. The pharmacy department was important, especially as the clinic was going to include some nurse prescribing, once final protocols were in place, and some medications with evidence to support their use were 'off licence' such as ketamine. Laboratory staff and the clinical measurement department were also informed of the proposal and their views sought. Based on the results of the initial examination, patient history and previous screening, additional tests would sometimes be required to determine the nature and extent of a neuropathy and these might include computed tomography (CT scan), magnetic resonance imaging, electromyography, nerve conduction velocity, nerve biopsy or skin biopsy. Although the relevant medical consultant would normally undertake the request of these tests, I might recommend one of them following a patient's assessment in the clinic.

As some patients would be commenced on a trial of opioids, the views of the substance misuse services would have been useful, but in the initial phase we did not make special contact as we already had a good working relationship with the substance misuse team established by the Acute Pain Service. We did not at the time contact any of the local company occupation health schemes either, but if a neuropathic pain service is to develop in primary care, having a system of contacting local employer health teams and liaising with social services may also have been useful.

Developing a business plan

Apart from making contact with key stakeholders, a business plan was the second most important requirement and something I did not have much experience of. Obtaining as much help as possible with this was very important as the rationale had to appear clear and focused, the outcomes realistic and the costings as accurate as possible. Obtaining a fighting fund was also crucial and in our case we were able to obtain a small start-up fund from a pharmaceutical company. This source of funding is controversial today, but we obtained a grant with no strings attached and in no way did the pharmaceutical company attempt to influence how the clinics were developed, the treatment algorithms designed or prescribing policy implemented. In hindsight, a trust/primary care trust (PCT) agreed funding stream would have helped to secure the future of the clinics beyond the initial pilot phase, but we were keen to get started, so began with just the initial grant.

It would have been shrewd and politic to have developed an accurate cost–benefit analysis but at the time obtaining meaningful data was just too difficult. However, a study published subsequently in 2007 appears to confirm that a shift in the locus of care of painful neuropathies from secondary care pain clinics to primary care may result in substantial cost savings to the health care system (Berger *et al.* 2007). We undertook an initial audit of patients referred during a 6-month trial period, which confirmed the extent of the problems patients faced and in fact indicated the possibility of reducing some of the prescribing costs as inappropriate or ineffective medications were discontinued. The data included a time to diagnosis of the pain and the impact and efficacy of current treatment. Most patients had no understanding of the diagnosis of painful diabetic neuropathy; they did not know what this was or the implications for treatment. We tried to evaluate the patient's journey to help develop a sound rationale for service development in the future. The goal being to include local patients, an early referral, clinical diagnosis and access to evidence-based treatment.

Assessment tools

For assessment we proposed to use the LANSS neuropathic pain assessment tool and the Brief Pain Inventory. For alternative tools designed for neuropathic pain assessment, see Table 4.1. Although at the time we did not include assessment tools specifically for depression, fear avoidance beliefs, disability and loss of function, etc., having tools available that have been designed to assess these is a useful strategy. Comprehensive assessment can help to identify, at the earliest possible opportunity, those patients at risk of significant psychological comorbidity that can impact on the success or failure of treatment strategies. However, I did not want the first consultation to be a form-filling exercise. Examples of a range of very useful and validated assessment tools currently available include the Hospital Anxiety and Depression Scale, which, despite its name, has been validated for use in primary care. The following were developed for people suffering from chronic musculoskeletal pain but are examples of validated tools useful for identifying some of the barriers to improving function and relieving distress: Fear Avoidance Beliefs Questionnaire (Waddell *et al.* 1993), Distress Risk Assessment Method (Main *et al.* 1992) and the SF-36, which is useful as a measure to assess physical and social functioning (Ware & Sherbourne 1992).

The proposed outcomes in the final business plan included the following:

- Reduced hospital admission – neuropathy accounts for more hospitalisations than all other diabetic complications combined. Twenty-eight percent of patients with microvascular complications developed neuropathy (Williams *et al.* 2002).
- Rapid evaluation of early-onset neuropathic pain – a high proportion of patients with idiopathic neuropathic pain have been shown to have impaired glucose tolerance (Singleton *et al.* 2001).

Table 4.1 Scales designed for neuropathic pain assessment

Instrument	Patient	Clinician	Suggested use	References
		Completed by		
NPS	X		Assessment of distinct qualities of neuropathic pain. Assessment of treatment effects	Galer and Jensen (1997)
LANSS		X	Identifying pain of predominantly neuropathic origin	Bennett (2001)
S-LANSS	X		Identifying pain of predominantly neuropathic origin	Bennett *et al.* (2005)
NPQ	X		Discrimination of neuropathic pain from non-neuropathic pain Assessment of treatment effects on neuropathic symptoms	Krause and Backonja (2003)
NPQ – short form	X		Screening of neuropathic pain	Backonja and Krause (2003)
NPSI	X		Assessment of distinct dimensions of neuropathic pain. Assessment of treatment effects	Bouhassira *et al.* (2004)
D4		X	Discrimination of neuropathic pain from non-neuropathic pain	Bouhassira *et al.* (2005)
D4-Interview	X		Screening of neuropathic pain	Bouhassira *et al.* (2005)
ID Pain	X		Screening of neuropathic pain	Portenoy (2006)
Pain DETECT	X		Screening a neuropathic component in low back pain	Freynhagen *et al.* (2006)

Taken from Hansson and Haanpaac (2007)

- Improved use of appropriate pharmacological strategies.
- A resulting reduction in patients remaining on inappropriate or ineffective medication.
- A reduction in side effects associated with medication.
- Improved functional status and quality of life.
- Improved personal knowledge and coping strategies.
- Ultimately, a decreased use of health care resources, leading to better-informed patients able to take responsibility for their ongoing pain management strategies and treatment goals.

For a breakdown of start-up costs and proposed funding streams, see the copy of the business plan in Appendix 1. Initially there was to be no impact on pharmacy costs as prescribing would remain in primary care.

In developing the business plan we also gave example documents with key features and their relevance to support the changes such as 'A health service of all the talents' (DH 2000), 'Agenda for change' (DH 2004), 'Saving lives: our healthier nation' (DH 1999), 'The expert patient: a new approach to chronic disease management for the 21st century' (DH 2001) and 'Working together for better diabetes care' (DH 2007).

The final part of the business plan recognised the importance of governance issues such as the Nursing and Midwifery Council's (2006) knowledge and skills framework, relevant qualifications, additional training needs of the practitioner, prescribing qualifications, access to medical consultation and implications for clinical supervision.

Although at the time we began the clinic only a limited number of evidenced-based algorithms for the management of neuropathic pain had been published and these had been developed predominantly in the USA, it was important to have a locally agreed protocol for treatment. More recent treatment algorithms are now available devised by clinicians from the UK, which reflect commonly prescribed medications, supported by more robust evidence. For example, an integrated care pathway developed specifically for the primary care management of neuropathic pain has been published by Bennett *et al.* (2006) as well as guidelines developed for Northern Ireland by the Clinical Resource Efficiency Support Team (CREST) (2008). Unfortunately, consistency appears to be the problem when selecting first-, second- and third-line drug treatments in all the guidelines and algorithms currently published (Finnerup *et al.* 2005; Dworkin *et al.* 2007; Moulin *et al.* 2007; Attal *et al.* 2006).

The challenges and reality

The clinic ran for 18 months and the next and most logical phase was taking it into primary care. Although developing and running these clinics proved challenging, I was privileged to spend many hours with some courageous and resourceful patients. I undertook an evaluation of the service at 6 months and at 1 year and what came across overwhelmingly was the gratitude of patients who had been given the opportunity to discuss their symptoms. A new patient had a 1-hour consultation, although in hindsight 1.5 hours would have been preferable. This time enabled them to discuss their pain, which had been to almost all of them, completely unexplained and a source of overwhelming distress. I was also able to explore some of the impact of their pain on their families, their attempts to retain and function in their jobs, their social lives and numerous other issues. Many expressed relief in knowing that they were not alone simply by the fact that there was now a clinic specifically for what one patient termed his 'invisible' pain. Not one patient I encountered had any idea what neuropathic pain was and their relief was palpable when I was able to explain to them just why they experienced, in many cases severe pain especially in their hands and feet, when everything looked 'normal'. Most patients had felt completely disbelieved by work colleagues, family and even in some cases by health care professionals.

For a considerable number of patients just one appointment was all they needed. The majority did not want to take medication on a long-term basis but were very pleased to know what was available and how it may work. Some patients needed to have their medications adjusted, either titrated up or replaced with an alternative if little or no benefit had been experienced. A significant number of patients had multiple medications discontinued altogether as they had proved totally ineffective. However, because they had been 'prescribed' in some instances, the medications had been taken for years seemingly without regular review. A few patients who had tried both antidepressants and anticonvulsants unsuccessfully were commenced on a trial of opioids. This was in the form of oral morphine for titration and then a slow release preparation for maintenance of pain control if they experienced an acceptable response. Oxycodone was usually recommended for the more elderly patients or for those who had a poor experience with morphine. Patients commencing on an opioid trial were followed up by telephone and a subsequent appointment. They were also given copies of the British Pain Society information for patients leaflet (British Pain Society 2004a). Significant numbers obtained some benefit from low doses taken twice a day, at night only or reserved for when pain became particularly distressing. Patients were warned to be patient as titration of medications for neuropathic pain can take time and optimal pain relief is often only obtained using polypharmacy.

Many patients were able to make the link between increasing stress, poor sleeping and painful flares, which made the inclusion of non-pharmacological strategies such as learning to relax, taking time out and improving sleeping habits useful. In published studies the most common management strategy was the use of conventional medications, often associated with poor effectiveness, but many found resting or retreating helpful (Closs *et al.* 2007). In this study by Closs, patients exhibited repeated cycles of seeking help to manage pain, being unsuccessful and then repeating the cycles again. Some had tried to accept their pain but found that there was insufficient psychological, social, emotional and practice support to allow them to do this successfully. An example of a case history to help illustrate working with patients to obtain a realistic and achievable goal is described in the case study given in Box 4.1. I undertook an assessment and we had a long talk about how she could continue in her job and control her pain better. It transpired that because of her high levels of responsibility and the impact this had on her during term time, her glycaemic control was not as good as it

---

Box 4.1 Case study of neuropathic pain.

Mrs M was a very senior teacher at a large comprehensive. She was an extremely stoic character but was finding the increasing pain in her feet, having a huge impact on her ability to carry out her job to her satisfaction. Standing for any length of time was becoming more difficult as her pain increased, but if she took amitriptyline 25 mg, which had been prescribed for her at night, she felt sedated and un-refreshed in the morning. She had undertaken a trial of several anticonvulsants, including gabapentin and pregabalin, but again she was left feeling sedated for what she felt was little improvement in her pain control. Unfortunately, she had also experienced some weight gain on anticonvulsants and this she found completely unacceptable. She was at her wits end and felt that she was facing no alternative but to retire on ill-health grounds. Something she had desperately tried to avoid since developing painful diabetic neuropathy, some 8 years previously.

should be. I explained that this could impact on her pain and she confirmed that she would be far more vigilant in the future. We discussed various options and came up with the following plan.

She would try capsaicin cream on her feet to see if she could obtain any pain relief with a topical medication. She would also try regular paracetamol 1 g for just 72 hours. Although the data on paracetamol for neuropathic pain are not impressive, some patients do seem to derive a little benefit with minimal side effects. If both these strategies failed, she would then try to reintroduce amitriptyline, which she felt had certainly helped with her sleep, but this time she would take it with an evening meal instead of just before going to bed and at a reduced dose of 10 mg. As she was very reluctant to undergo another trial of anticonvulsants, it was suggested that she trial a strong opioid during the impending half-term. This was so she would not have to drive and if she felt a little sedated, she could stay at home and monitor her analgesia without the stresses of a demanding job.

At her next visit, neither the capsaicin nor paracetamol had been of any great benefit, but to her delight the trial of oral morphine at a dose of just 20 mg reduced her pain intensity from an average of 7/10 down to a manageable 3/10. Also the low-dose amitriptyline at just 10 mg had enhanced her ability to go to sleep and reduced the impact of night-time pain, but she still felt unrefreshed in the morning. The tricyclic antidepressant was changed to a low dose of nortryptyline, which ultimately suited her better. Once term began, Mrs M only used morphine very frugally and only when pain at night or during the weekends was particularly troublesome. As she said, knowing what was causing her pain, being far more diligent in managing her diabetes, getting a better night's sleep and just having morphine there if she needed it left her feeling better able to cope with the pain. She was happy to be discharged on no further medication and with just an SOS appointment if she needed it.

Although I felt the clinics were filling a gap in patient care, it was not always straightforward. I would sometimes get referrals from patients who had already done the rounds of the pain clinics and pain management programmes, but had not come to terms with their pain and were still seeking somebody to 'cure' them. Having very clear referral criteria might have overcome this problem. During the time I was undertaking the clinics, despite being a prescriber, the individual hospital protocol for nurse prescribers was not completed, so the prescribing of medication trials was left to patient's GPs. This inevitably built in a delay and meant patients had to visit their GP a day or two after the clinics to have a new regime commenced or to have medication doses adjusted, and this was far from ideal.

GPs were informed that their patient had attended a nurse-led neuropathic pain clinic and the strategies that had been discussed. This was forwarded to them in the form of an electronic letter on the day of the clinic. See Appendix 3 for an example of a typical letter, which reflects in many cases the desire for an explanation and medication options, even though quite often patients then declined to take these. About half the patients seen did not want to take further medication but just wanted to know what was going on and what they could expect in the future. Overall, the GPs appeared to be very supportive and none of them refused a patient the medications suggested even when this included a trial of an opioid.

Following my retirement I took a 6-month break and then hoped to resume the clinics on a fortnightly basis. It proved somewhat difficult to keep up appropriate referrals when I no longer had a full-time presence within the hospital and delays with organising a part-time casual contract meant the 6 months became nearly a year. By then I felt the momentum had gone and I left the NHS completely in 2005 to devote my part-time hours to the development of web-based postgraduate education strategies. There were things we did not get right but I certainly feel that the model of a nurse-led neuropathic pain clinic in primary care could work and provide tremendous benefit to patients with this distressing condition as well as helping to reduce the burden on hard-pressed GPs and pain clinics.

Evaluation of the service

Evaluation of a new service and an audit trail are a major part of the culture of the NHS today. Audit and research data from around the world can highlight the problems associated with a wide range of neuropathic pain but particularly painful diabetic neuropathy and post-herpetic neuralgia. Audit and evaluation of the clinics were undertaken on a regular basis, with patient feedback obtained using the audit and evaluation strategies recommended in 'A practical guide to the provision of chronic pain services for adults in primary care' (British Pain Society 2004b). First and foremost the audit data were able to allay initial fears that there would be a vast increase in prescribing costs. This did not seem to be the case and many patients actually had ineffective prescribed medications discontinued or had their medications streamlined rather than remaining on a range of similar drugs. Audit was also able to show that patients did not come back for numerous clinic visits. During the first visit of 1 hour we were able to explore many issues and discuss strategies with the specific goal of putting the patient in control, armed with improved knowledge, with booklets and websites to view if appropriate, and a treatment regime to follow as necessary.

Follow-up appointments were made only when patients particularly requested these, they were undertaking a trial of opioids, their care was especially challenging or it was deemed they may benefit from further psychological input. The reality at the time was that although access to the specialist pain clinic psychologist would have been the ideal, local psychology input was already at capacity. Despite my attempts I did not have the knowledge and skills to undertake any more than very rudimentary psychological support, but listening and empathy are skills we can all develop. Directing patients to the expert patient programme and various charitable self-help organisations such as the Neuropathy Trust proved beneficial for some. Training for myself in cognitive behavioural therapy would certainly have been a great advantage and something I intended to explore further at a later date. It would also have been an advantage to be able to refer particularly complex patients to a clinical psychologist or into a pain management programme but availability and cost issues meant this was not a reality at the time. Data were also analysed from the Brief Pain Inventory. Although a significant reduction in pain at follow-up was rarely achieved, improvements were seen in sleep, function and mood.

Justifying the advanced nursing contribution

Although many nurse specialists now run clinics for a wide range of conditions, I feel the development of a neuropathic pain clinic appropriately reflects advanced nursing practice. Neuropathic pain is hugely complex and not fully understood; the diagnosis is not always straightforward and rarely will pain respond to simple analgesia. Many medical staff display scant knowledge or experience of managing this complex pain and the inevitable psychological fallout from the symptoms of intractable neuropathic pain. Research indicates that so far the medications prescribed by non-specialists are generally inappropriate, such as amitriptyline in the older patient, or anticonvulsant medication rarely titrated upwards beyond a low starting dose.

For nurses to undertake these clinics, some advanced education in pain management would be required and ideally they would need to be a prescriber in primary care to optimise cost–benefit. There are now a significant number of specialist pain nurses who have undergone a degree in this subject and have been closely involved in the care of patients in pain for many years. Nurses may be in a better position to devote the time needed for the care of these complex patients and their needs. Once the clinics are established, they also provide an important opportunity to pass on acquired skills and knowledge to colleagues and peers. Therefore, advanced practice nurses would need to be comfortable with publishing results and disseminating these as widely as possible. They may also be called upon to become more closely involved in the pain education of other health care professionals.

Conclusions

Initiating a nurse-led neuropathic pain clinic requires a great deal of support from physicians, administrators, nurses, podiatrists and clerical staff as well as the endorsement from the relevant trust boards, irrespective of whether the clinic is designed to run in primary or secondary care. Evaluating the impact these clinics may have on patients, their families, staff, health care professionals and even perhaps employers provides the evidence to support their development and expansion when positive outcomes prove achievable. The cost implications do not have to be particularly significant as benefit in some cases may be illustrated by more effective use of medication, improved patient care and a possible reduction in patient access to their GP or specialist pain clinics. Although my particular clinic was in its infancy with issues that needed to be addressed, I firmly believe that the model provided a basis, which could be built on and adapted in the future.

It is important to make use of the recent advances in treatments particularly as we expand our knowledge in the field of pharmacogenetics (Gilron *et al.* 2002; Stamer *et al.* 2005). Our understanding of the influence of genotype on pharmacokinetics and pharmacodynamics will enable us to target effective medications, and as science unravels the complexities associated with the 'drivers' of neuropathic pain, the future is also looking more promising. In addition, an expanding knowledge of the 'talking therapies' will provide more meaningful psychological support. Working with patients and having access to the professional skills of a multidisciplinary pain management team only for patients who do not respond to first-, second- or even third-line treatments would ensure that time is not wasted on referring patients for whom a comprehensive assessment, a medication regime change, simple psychological therapies and personal education may suffice.

Appendix 1: Original business plan

Development of a nurse led clinic for the management of painful neuropathy

Department/Unit	Medicine	Project Proposers
Funding Required	£.	Drs . . . .
		Nurse . . . .
Funding Sources	The Modernisation Agenda Budget, Industry sponsorship & Charitable Trusts for start up monies	PCT + on going support from Industrial sponsorship, Charitable Trusts & Clinical Trials

1   Bid Summary

Patients consistently identify pain management as a key issue in health care. The following details how senior nursing staff with special expertise in pain management within The. . . . . NHS Trust Hospital could undertake a nurse led clinic under the supervision of a Lead Consultant within the Diabetic Centre and The Pain Clinic for the management and evaluation of patients with chronically painful neuropathies.

This is set out in the context of initiatives/policies such as the consultative document

- 'A Health Service of all the Talents' (DH 2000), Agenda for Change (DH 2004), Saving lives: our healthier nation (DH 1999)
- The expert patient: a new approach to chronic disease management for the 21st century, http://www.dh.gov.uk/en/Publicationsandstatistics/Publications/Publications PolicyAndGuidance/DH_4006801
- The NHS plan. A plan for investment. A plan for reform, http://www.dh.gov.uk/en/Publicationsandstatistics/Publications/PublicationsPolicyAndGuidance/DH_4002960 The National Service Frameworks for the Elderly & Diabetes. (DH 2007) Working together for better diabetes care. http://www.dh.gov.uk/en/Publicationsandstatistics/Publications/PublicationsPolicy AndGuidance/DH_074702
- The Principles of Integrated Service Transformation, http://www.isip.nhs.uk/

2   Project Rationale – Aims/Objectives

The development of a Nurse Led Clinic for the management of painful neuropathies would complement the current pain management services such as the Acute Pain Service and Chronic Pain Clinic. It would also provide an excellent opportunity to enhance the liaison currently being developed with the local Primary Care Trusts. The Clinic will assist patients to improve coping strategies and pain control using a range of pharmacological and non pharmacological therapies based on the latest available evidence and where possible, following an agreed algorithm or care pathway.

The clinic will employ comprehensive assessment of pain intensity as well as the impact of pain on patients' functional status and daily activities. Other issues such as sleep disturbance and fatigue will be assessed, as well as psychosocial factors such as depression, anxiety and fear avoidance. The clinic will provide the opportunity for erroneous beliefs and misconceptions to be discussed and addressed.

The clinic will also enable evaluation of pharmacological strategies including efficacy, duration of action, and side effects following an agreed algorithm. This will include the use of simple and strong analgesia, tricyclic antidepressants, anti-convulsants, antiarrhythmics, topical medications and other adjuvant medications deemed appropriate.

Non pharmacological strategies will also be available such as a trial of TENS and behaviour change skills. Behaviour change skills (BCS) are seen as important in influencing health status. BCS are a combination of psychological approaches, which can be applied in traditional clinical settings and are evidence based. These are 'Motivational Approaches' (adapted from Motivational Interviewing) and 'Cognitive Behavioural Approaches' (adapted from Cognitive Behavioural Therapy).

Patient information sheets such as *Opioid Medication for Chronic Painful Conditions* produced by the British Pain Society www.painsociety.org will be used for any patients those treatment may include a trial of strong opioids. Additional information sheets will be developed to accompany any other pharmacological strategies that are commenced. A care plan/patient held diary that informs the patient and their GP of their treatment with further options to be considered listed according to strength of supporting evidence. These will be itemised in the diary to improve evaluation of strategies, enhance communication and to avoid the reuse of medications already deemed to have failed or which have contributed to unacceptable side effects.

3   Links/Relevance to National Priorities for Health, Education and Training

This is set out in the context of initiatives/policies discussed out in the consultative documents previously listed.

4   Links with Local Strategic Priorities

National Service Framework for Elderly Care, Mental Health & Diabetes

5   Expected Outcomes

- Reduced hospital admission – neuropathy accounts for more hospitalizations than all other diabetic complications combined. 28% of patients with micro vascular complications develop neuropathy (Williams *et al.* 2002)
- Rapid evaluation of early onset neuropathic pain – a high proportion of patients with idiopathic neuropathic pain have been shown to have impaired glucose tolerance (Singleton *et al.* 2001)
- Improved use of appropriate pharmacological strategies
- A resulting reduction in patients remaining on inappropriate or ineffective medication
- A reduction in side effects associated with medication
- Improved functional status and quality of life
- Improved personal knowledge and coping strategies
- Ultimately, a decreased use of health care resources leading to better informed patients able to take responsibility for their ongoing pain management strategies and treatment goals.

6   Collaboration, Multi Professional/Inter-Disciplinary Elements [where appropriate]

This initiative would help to improve pain management within Primary & Secondary Care via the patient held diary (with data duplicated in electronic patient records) informing a wide range of health care professionals current strategies being trialed, potential side effects and any benefits perceived so far. Goals could be set to help patients achieve the best possible functional status and quality of life and these would be made explicit. By setting common goals and listing strategies previously tried or currently under review, patients would be assured that their pain is taken seriously, that there is a logical pathway to their care and all relevant health care professionals are informed. Much iatrogenic damage can occur when patients are prescribed ineffective or inappropriate medication, fail to have access to the latest evidence based treatment or appropriate treatment is delayed until pain has become intractable.

7   Evaluation Tool, Process for Sharing Results

Patients pain perception, quality of life issues, functional status and other psychosocial issues that may contribute to a poor pain outcome will be evaluated.
Results will be disseminated widely and written up for publication

8   Financial Breakdown, Project Timescale

Financial breakdown
Start up costs:

- Administration, secretarial support and stationary £ . . . .
- Cost for medical records and note retrieval £. . . . .
- Development of assessment and evaluation tools £. . . . .
- Development and printing of comprehensive information leaflets for patients £. . . . .
- Development and printing of patient held diaries £. . . . .
- Laptop for use by clinicians to store records of patient contact, audit data, results of evaluation and dissemination literature £. . . . .
- Outpatient hourly rate £. . . . .
- Practitioner hourly rate £. . . . .

Initially there will be no impact on pharmacy costs as prescribing will remain in primary care for the pilot project.

Total money sought for pilot of this project £. . . . .

Monies for this project will be sought from The Modernisation Agenda Budget, The Pharmaceutical Industry & Charitable Trusts. The project could be linked to the University Academic Centre in Practice and provide scope for the further education of health care professionals. In addition, a database of patients will become established who may be suitable/willing to undertake clinical trials for new therapy/medications as these are developed. This could provide a considerable source of additional funding.

Project Timescale

- We would be able to commence the first patient clinic in . . . . to run as a pilot for twelve months.
- After this time an evaluation of the service would be undertaken and if the initiative was deemed effective, an application for on going funding would be made to the PCT. This would include a sum of £. . . . . to support ongoing nursing involvement.
- On going pain management would ideally revert to the community following further education for Health Care Professionals facilitated by the Academic Centre in Practice and via the staff educated in the first wave of the community pain education project.

Contact Leads: Drs. . . . .
Nurse Consultant Pain Management . . . .
Lecturer Practitioner Pain Management . . . .

Appendix 2: Text of an open letter to all local general practitioners informing them of the proposal to commence a nurse-led clinic for painful diabetic neuropathy

Developing a nurse-led pain clinic for patients experiencing painful diabetic neuropathy

Neuropathic pain is caused by damage, disease or dysfunction within the nervous system. Unfortunately this type of pain is often refractory to conventional analgesic therapy, it is frequently persistent and does not resolve with time. As a consequence, it is experienced as a debilitating condition, with a bleak outlook that inevitably has a negative impact on the quality of patients' lives. Due to previous lack of evidence to support any therapeutic intervention and many misconceptions regarding possible treatment, the management of neuropathic pain has traditionally been poor.

There is no doubt that diabetes, through multiple pathophysiological mechanisms, is capable of causing several painful neuropathies and its management is therefore complex and time consuming. However, recent evidence is suggesting that if symptoms can be relieved early, then patients may experience improved outcomes in terms of reduced pain and enhanced quality of life.

The rapid growth of scientific research is offering us a better understanding of neuropathic pain. With this advancing understanding, evidence based strategies; both pharmacological and non-pharmacological are emerging. Specially trained nurses are in an excellent position to assist with the care of these complex patients and can offer an approach evaluating a full range of therapies through comprehensive assessment which helps to address issues such as expectation, rehabilitation, mobility, lifestyle, sleep, emotional impact and quality of life as well as pain control. This new initiative introducing a specialist pain nurse has been developed to enhance the traditional services offered by the diabetic management team.

Each patient will undergo a thorough assessment using a variety of pain assessment tools. Patients will be given information and education about the possible mechanism of their pain and how symptoms may be controlled. This may include the initiation and then on going monitoring of a range of pharmacological strategies to include tricyclic antidepressants, anticonvulsants, opioids and topical medications. Any patients commenced on any of these therapies would be followed up if necessary either at clinic or via a telephone review. Any opioid trial would follow the guidelines produced by the Pain Society on Opioids for Chronic Non-Maligant Pain and patients would be given a copy of the Pain Society's leaflet before making any decision to undertake this therapy. Their General Practitioner would be fully informed of any pharmacological intervention and in the case of an opioid trial their agreement for participation would be sought prior to initiation.

In addition to pharmacological strategies the emphasis would be on long term pain management, reinforced coping strategies and promotion of self-management. Patients would be treated as partners in their care whilst kept fully informed of their diagnosis and treatment options. They would also be made aware of expert patient programmes and relevant voluntary organisations.

Some of the key benefits that we hope to offer include; improving patients' knowledge and awareness, increasing mobility and thereby hopefully enhancing quality of life. We also intend to monitor and address issues of psychological morbidity, actively managing symptoms and providing telephone follow-up to enhance continuity of care. By encouraging patients to self-manage we hope to reduce the burden on health care providers. We will be able to act as an educational resource for clinical staff in both Primary and Secondary Care and we intend to apply for additional funding to help research this complex and distressing pain.

A Nurse Consultant or a lecturer practitioner in Pain Management will undertake initial clinics. Both have extensive experience within the field of pain management and are responsible for university multi-professional undergraduate and post-graduate pain education. The clinics will run alongside those of the Consultant Physician. Following a diagnosis of painful diabetic neuropathy patients will be offered a referral to the nurse led clinic. Patients will be fully informed that this is nurse led and given the opportunity to decline should they wish. The clinic will initially take place once per week and aim to see approximately 8 new and up to 8 follow up patients per month.

If this pilot is successful we would be happy to run further clinics with a view to transferring the service to Primary Care as and when future collaborative models evolve. The Pain Society and the Royal College of General Practitioners have endorsed five pledges to help people living with persistent pain. These include ensuring that the government, local NHS Trusts, and self-help groups prioritise effective management of persistent pain. The pledge also suggests NHS service providers and commissioners should work to adopt care pathways for people living with persistent pain across the primary, community and secondary care sectors.

The clinic will help to meet the governments' aim of increasing patient focused services, that develop nurses' roles and reduce the workload of junior doctors. The clinics will offer the added benefit of providing a platform for valuable interprofessional education and research.

Contact details

Appendix 3: Example of a typical letter to a general practitioner, at the time pregabalin was not available for prescription

Painful Diabetic Neuropathy Clinic
Diabetes Centre,

15th April 2004
cc. Dr. . . . . Medical Consultant

Dr. D. Bloggs
The Surgery
Town, County

Dear Dr.
Re: Mr C   Hospital No . . . . DOB

Today I saw Mr C for the first time at a Painful Diabetic Neuropathy Clinic we have established to run in conjunction with Dr. B's clinics. The following is a synopsis of my assessment and suggestions for a possible management strategy that may be appropriate for the future. Unfortunately Mr C experiences painful diabetic neuropathy in a stocking and glove distribution rating average pain intensity as 8/10.

Previous and current pain medication:
Amitriptyline 25 mg Some mild benefit but excessive sedation so discontinued
Gabapentin 600 mg bd Some relief from 'shock' type pains but sedation problematic and dose could not be increased due to renal insufficiency
Piroxicam some benefit
Voltarol no benefit
All NSAIDs have now been discontinued due to compromised renal function

Paracetamol 1 g	*no benefit*
Co-dydramol	*no benefit*
Tramadol	*no benefit*
Capsaicin cream	*no benefit and unpleasant*
TENS machine	*no benefit*

Ice pack some mild benefit

We had a long talk about his various options and one group of drugs he has not tried are strong opioids. Recent studies suggest these drugs can provide pain relief to some patients with painful neuropathy. Unfortunately the fact that Mr C.'s job involves driving, sedation is already problematic and he has renal problems make a trial of opioids more challenging. I have asked him to read the patient leaflet on 'Opioids for non malignant pain' produced by The British Pain Society who also provide prescriber information on www.britishpainsociety.org. He does not wish to try opioids at the current time but if you and he decide that a trail is appropriate, he should try a small dose of immediate release oral morphine over a weekend whilst he isn't at work or driving. If oral immediate release morphine confers any benefit and side effects are acceptable Mr C. should be converted to a slow release bd preparation based on his opioid requirement over 24 hours. Should his renal function continue to deteriorate, it would be worthwhile considering a change to either oxycontin or perhaps a fentanyl patch as neither of these drugs have clinically significant metabolites unlike morphine. Alternatively a burprenorphine patch may be a safer alternative as the drug is excreted via the liver.

For an opioid trail we would normally start at 10–30 mg oral morphine qds plus the same for breakthrough pain 3hrly prn. titrated up to effect or side effect. Given his compromised renal function I have given him additional advice about how to take these drugs more safely. He would not be able to drive for at least 7 hours after the last dose and not for 12 weeks if he were to be established on opioids long term. He has been advised to keep a pain diary to document any benefits/side effects should he choose this route. However, at present he is still very keen to work without a break and feels opioids may be something to consider at a future date if his pain begins to cause him greater distress. If this is the case I would be very happy for him to make a further appointment at the clinic for assessment and monitoring.

I have also supplied Mr C. with a booklet on neuropathic pain. We spent some time exploring some of the non-pharmacological strategies suggested in the booklet as well as the possibility of specialist pain clinic referral, which he declined for now. He feels these suggestions are helpful and we have left it that he can contact me for advice at any time.

Yours sincerely,
Nurse Consultant in Pain Management
Contact Tel No and Bleep No.

References

Attal, N., Cruccu, G., Haanpaa, M., Hansson, P., Jensen, T., Nurmikko, T., Sampaio, C., Sindrup, S., Wiffen, P., 2006. EFNS guidelines on pharmacological treatment of neuropathic pain. *European Journal of Neruology*, 13(11), 1153–1169.

Backonja, M., 2003. Defining neuropathic pain. *Anesthesia and Analgesia*, 97, 585–590.

Bennett, G., 1997. Neuropathic pain: an overview. In Borsook, K. (ed.), *Molecular Neurobiology of Pain*, pp. 109–113. Seattle: IASP Press.

Bennett, M., 2001. The LANSS Pain Scale: the Leeds assessment of neuropathic symptoms and signs. *Pain*, 92, 147–157.

Bennett, M., Simpson, K., Knaggs, R., Lloyd, S., Poole, H., Taylor, A., Kocan, M., Johnson, M., Archard, G., Baranidharan, G., Neuropathic Pain Advisory Groups, 2006. Neuropathic pain integrated care pathway evidence base. Prepared in association with and supported by NAPP Pharmaceuticals Ltd.

Bennett, M., Smith, B., Torrance, N., Potter, J., 2005. The S-LANNS score for identifying of predominantly neuropathic origin: validation for use in clinical and postal research. *The Journal of Pain*, 6(3), 149–158.

Berger, A., Kramarz, P., Kopperud, G., Edelsberg, J., Oster, G., 2007. Economic impact of shifting the locus of care for neuropathic pain from specialists to general practitioners. *The European Journal of Health Economics*, 8(3), 245–251.

Bouhassira, D., Attal, N., Fermanian, J., Alchaar, H., Gautron, M., Masquelier, E., Rostaing, S., Lanteri-Minet, M., Collin, E., Grisart, J., Boureau, F., 2004. Development and validation of the neuropathic pain symptom inventory. *Pain*, 108, 248–257.

Bouhassira, D., Attal, N., Alchaar, H., Boureau, F., Brochet, B., Bruxelle, J., Cunin, G., Fermanian, J., Ginies, P., Grun-Overdyking, A., Jafari-Schluep, H., Lantéri-Minet, M., Laurent, B., Mick, G., Serrie, A., Valade, D., Vicaut, E., 2005. Comparison of pain syndromes associated with nervous or somatic lesions and development of a new neuropathic pain diagnostic questionnaire (DN4). *Pain*, 114, 29–36.

British Pain Society, 2004a. Opioid medicines for persistent pain information for patients. Available at http://www.britishpainsociety.org/patient_publications.htm [accessed 20 February 2009].

British Pain Society, 2004b. A practical guide to the provision of chronic pain services for adults in primary are. Available at http://www.britishpainsociety.org/NAPP_RESOURCEPACK.pdf [accessed 20 February 2009].

Cavenagh, J., Good, P., Ravenscroft, P., 2006. Neuropathic pain: are we out of the woods yet? *Internal Medicine Journal*, 36, 251–255.

Closs, S., Staples, V., Reid, I., Bennett, M., Briggs, M., 2007. Managing the symptoms of neuropathic pain: an exploration of patients' experiences. *Journal of Pain and Symptom Management*, 34(4), 422–433.

Davies, H., Crombie, I., Macrae, W., 1994. Cited in Harden, N., Cohen, M., 2003. Unmet needs in the management of neuropathic pain. *Journal of Pain and Symptom Management*, 25(5S), S12–S17.

Department of Health, 1999. Saving lives our healthier nation. Available at http://www.dh. gov.uk/en/Publicationsandstatistics/Publications/PublicationsPolicyAndGuidance/DH_ 4008701 [accessed 25 February 2009].

Department of Health, 2000. A health service of all the talents. Available at http://www.dh. gov.uk/en/Publicationsandstatistics/Publications/PublicationsPolicyAndGuidance/DH_ 4007967 [accessed 25 February 2009].

Department of Health, 2001. The expert patient: a new approach to chronic disease management. Available at http://www.dh.gov.uk/en/Publicationsandstatistics/Publications/ PublicationsPolicyandGuidance/DH_4006801 [accessed 25 February 2009].

Department of Health, 2004. Agenda for change. Available at http://www.dh.gov.uk/en/ Managingyourorganisation/Humanresourcesandtraining/Modernisingpay/Agendaforchange/ index.htm [accessed 25 February 2009].

Department of Health, 2006. *Our Health, Our Care, Our Say: A New Direction for Community Services*. London: The Stationery Office.

Department of Health, 2007. Working together for better diabetes care. Available at http:// www.dh.gov.uk/en/Publicationsandstatistics/Publications/PublicationsPolicyAndGuidance/ DH_074702 [accessed 25 February 2009].

Dworkin, R., 2002. An overview of neuropathic pain: syndromes, symptoms, signs, and several mechanisms. *The Clinical Journal of Pain*, 18(6), 343–349.

Dworkin, R., O'Connor, A., Backonja, M., Farrar, J., Finnerup, N., Jensen, T., 2007. Pharma-cologic management of neuropathic pain: evidence-based recommendations. *Pain*, 132(3), 237–251.

Finnerup, N., Johannesen, I., Sindrup, S., Bach, F., Jensen, T., 2001. Pain and dysesthesia in patients with spinal cord injury: a postal survey. *Spinal Cord*, 39, 256–262.

Finnerup, N., Otto, M., McQuay, H., Jensen, T., Sindrup, S., 2005. Algorithm for neuropathic pain treatment: an evidence based proposal. *Pain*, 118(3), 289–305.

Fishbain, D., 1999. Approaches to treatment decisions for psychiatric co morbidity in the management of the chronic pain patients. *Emergency Medicine Clinics of North America*, 83, 737–760, vii.

Freynhagen, R., Baron, R., Gockel, U., Tolle, T., 2006. painDETECT: a new screening ques-tionnaire to identify neuropathic components in patients with back pain. *Current Medical Research and Opinion*, 22, 1911–1920.

Galer, B., Jensen, M., 1997. Development and preliminary validation of a pain measure specific to neuropathic pain. *Neurology*, 48, 332–338.

Gilron, I., Bailey, J., Weaver, D., Houlden, R., 2002. Patients' attitudes and prior treatments in neuropathic pain: a pilot study. *Pain Research and Management*, 7, 199–203.

Gore, M., Brandenburg, N., Hoffman, D., Tai, K., Stacey, B., 2006. Burden of illness in painful diabetic peripheral neuropathy: the patients' perspectives. *Journal of Pain*, 7(12), 892–900.

Gustorff, B., Dorner, T., Likar, R., Grisold, W., Lawrence, K., Schwarz, F., Rieder, A., 2008. Prevalence of self-reported neuropathic pain and impact on quality of life: a prospective representative survey. *Acta Anaesthesiologica Scandinavica*, 52(1), 132–136.

Hans, G., Masquelier, E., De Cock, P., 2007. The diagnosis and management of neuropathic pain in daily practice in Belgium: an observational study. *BMC Public Health*, 7 (147), 170.

Available at http://www.biomedcentral.com/content/pdf/1471–2458-7–170.pdf [accessed 20 February 2009].

Hansson, P., Haanpaac, M., 2007. Diagnostic work-up of neuropathic pain: computing using questionnaires or examining the patient? *European Journal of Pain*, 11(4), 367–369.

Harden, N., Cohen, M., 2003. Unmet needs in the management of neuropathic pain. *Journal of Pain and Symptom Management*, 25(5S), S12–S17.

Kawena, M., Omori, Y., Katayama, S., Kawakami, M., Suzuki, Y., Takahashi, K., Takemura, Y., Nagata, N., Hiratsuka, A., Matsuzaki, F., Kanazawa, Y., Akanuma, Y., 2001. A questionnaire for neurological symptoms in patients with diabetes – cross sectional multicentre study in Saitama Prefecture, Japan. *Diabetes Research and Clinical Practice*, 54(1), 41–47.

Krause, S., Backonja, M., 2003. Development of a Neuropathic Pain Questionnaire. *The Clinical Journal of Pain*, 19(5), 306–314.

Main, C., Wood, P., Hollis, S., Spanswick, C., Waddell, G., 1992. The distress and risk assessment method. A simple patient classification to identify distress and evaluate the risk of poor outcome. *Spine*, 17(1), 42–52.

McDermott, A., Toelle, T., Rowbotham, D., Schaefer, C., Dukes, E., 2006. The burden of neuropathic pain: results from a cross-sectional survey. *European Journal of Pain*, 10(2), 127–153.

Merskey, H., Bogduk, N., 1994. *Classification of Chronic Pain – Description of Chronic Pain Syndromes and Definitions of Pain Terms*, 2nd edn. Seattle: IASP Press.

Morritt Taub, L., Redeker, N., 2008. Sleep disorders, glucose regulation and type 2 diabetes. *Biological Research for Nursing*, 9(3), 231–243.

Moulin, D., Clark, A., Gilron, I., Ware, M., Watson, C., Sessle, B., Coderre, T., Morley-Forster, P., Stinson, J., Boulanger, A., Peng, P., Finley, G., Taenzer, P., Squire, P., Dion, D., Cholkan, A., Gilani, A., Gordon, A., Henry, J., Jovey, R., Lynch, M., Mailis-Gagnon, A., Panju, A., Rollman, G., Velly, A., 2007. Pharmacological management of chronic neuropathic pain – consensus statement and guidelines from the Canadian Pain Society. *Pain Research and Management*, 12(1), 13–21.

Nursing and Midwifery Council, 2006. Advanced nursing practice update – 4. Available at http://www.nmc-uk.org/aArticle.aspx?ArticleID=2038 [accessed 20 February 2009].

Orza, F., Boswell, M., Rosenberg, S., 2000. Neuropathic pain: review of mechanisms and pharmacologic management. *NeuroRehabilitation*, 14, 15–23.

Portenoy, R., 2006. Development and testing of a neuropathic pain screening questionnaire: ID pain. *Current Medical Research and Opinion*, 22, 1555–1565.

Richeimer, S., Bajwa, Z., Kahraman, S., Bernard, A., Warfield, C., 1997. Utilization patterns of tricyclic antidepressants in a multidisciplinary clinic: a survey. *The Clinical Journal of Pain*, 13, 324–329.

Singleton, J., Smith, A., Bromberg, M., 2001. Painful sensory polyneuropathy associated with impaired glucose tolerance. *Muscle and Nerve*, 24 (9), 1225–1228.

Stamer, U., Bayerer, B., Stuber, F., 2005. Genetics and variability in opioid response. *European Journal of Pain*, 9, 131–135.

Taylor, R., 2006. Epidemiology of refractory neuropathic pain. *Pain Practice*, 6(1), 22–26.

The Clinical Resource Efficiency Support Team (CREST), 2008. Guidelines on the management of neuropathic pain. Available at http://www.crestni.org.uk/crest_-management_of_neuropathic_pain_guidelines-2.pdf [accessed 20 February 2009].

Torrance, N., Smith, B., Bennett, M., *et al.*, 2005. The epidemiology of neuropathic pain in the community: preliminary results from a general population survey. *Poster Presented at the Annual Scientific Meeting of the British Pain Society*. Edinburgh, UK, 8–11 March.

Turk, D., Gatchel, R., 2002. *Psychological Approaches to Pain Management: A Practitioner's Handbook*. New York: Guildford Press.

Waddell, G., Newton, M., Henderson, I., Somerville, D., Main, C., 1993. A Fear Avoidance Beliefs Questionnaire (FABG) and the role of fear-avoidance beliefs in chronic low back pain and disability. *Pain*, 52, 57–68.

Ware, J., Sherbourne, C., 1992. The MOS 36-item short-form health survey (SF-36) I. Conceptual framework and item selection. *Medical Care*, 30, 473–483.

Williams, R., Van Gaal, L., Lucioni, C., 2002. Assessing the impact of complications on the costs of type II diabetes. *Diabetologia*, 45(7), S13–S17.

Zelman, D., Brandenburg, N., Gore, M., 2006. Sleep impairment in patients with painful diabetic peripheral neuropathy. *The Clinical Journal of Pain*, 22(8), 681–685.

Chapter 5
Nurse-led strategies to improve patient safety in acute pain management

Felicia Cox

Introduction

Advances in delivery technology and an expansion in the choice of analgesia preparations have evoked rapid changes in acute pain management in the hospital setting over the last two decades. This increase in technology and enlarged formulary contribute to an increase in the risk of medication-related adverse events (MRAEs). More than 4.2 million surgical procedures are performed in England per annum (Department of Health [DH] 2009). This means that on average 1 in 12 people had some form of surgical intervention and thus were at risk of an adverse MRAE. Royston and Cox (2003) explored patient concerns related to safety, outcome and comfort. They concluded that many patients worry that they will not wake up after surgery, will experience intraoperative awareness, suffer mental impairment or will have unrelieved nausea, vomiting and pain.

Analgesia in the hospital setting has been the subject of the National Patient Safety Agency (NPSA) guidance constituting 1 of 11 published Rapid Response reports and 3 of the 10 Patient Safety Alerts. Two additional early Patient Safety Alerts focused on standardising methotrexate prescribing and administration. The NPSA (www.npsa.nhs.uk) is responsible in England and Wales for the central recording and reporting of adverse incidents via the National Reporting and Learning System. A patient safety incident is defined as any unintended or unexpected incident which could have or did lead to harm for one or more patients receiving NHS care (NPSA 2008). Incidents can be reported locally within an NHS Trust by a member of staff or directly to the NPSA on their website (www.npsa.nhs.uk/nrls/reporting/) by an NHS employee, a patient or the public.

Incidents are analysed and although no two incidents are identical, similarities and patterns are identified and guidance issued where necessary. Over 2.7 million reports have been received by the NPSA over the last 5 years, leading to the development of the 21 published guidance documents.

In addition to NHS trusts undertaking continual reviews of care and adverse events to enhance patient safety and reduce annual premiums for the NHS Litigation Authority, a National Patient Safety First has been established (www.patientsafetyfirst.nhs.uk).

Media exposure

Adverse events related to inpatient medicine administration via neuraxial routes that have resulted in patient disability and death have resulted in unprecedented media coverage over the last 5 years. The inadvertent administration of vincristine into the intrathecal space rather than as an intravenous injection for the treatment of leukaemia has been reported more than 55 times worldwide. Intrathecal vincristine results in either death or paralysis. The death of a patient in 2001 (Timesonline 2003) led to the development of guidelines from the DH for the administration of chemotherapy. This document is currently under review in response to a more recent circular that relates specifically to the administration of intrathecal chemotherapy (DH 2008).

An analgesia-related story covered by the press was that of a television actress who was awarded a £5 million settlement after developing an abscess following epidural analgesia for fractured ribs and a resultant pneumothorax in 2004 (Timesonline 2008a). The amount of the record settlement reflected what the NHS Trust responsible described as 'shortcomings in her care'.

Also in 2004 a theatre nurse in labour received an inadvertent intravenous infusion of the local anaesthetic bupivacaine in the hospital where she worked. Bupivacaine is known to induce profound disturbances in cardiac rhythm and contractility (Astra Zeneca 2005). This infusion resulted in fatal cardiotoxicity and neurotoxicity. In 2008 her death was deemed by the coroner and jury as unlawful killing (Timesonline 2008b). This was the first verdict of unlawful killing against an NHS hospital. In the light of these events and the potential of serious harm or even patient death, it was important to try and reduce the risks associated with neuraxial administration of medicines including analgesia.

Injectable medicines

Injectable medicines are responsible for nearly a quarter of the annual total of medication incidents reported through the National Reporting and Learning System with approximately 800 reports per month. During an 18-month period (January 2005 to June 2006) injectable medicines were responsible for 25 patient deaths and 28 patients experienced severe harm (NPSA 2007a). Injectable opioid medicines for acute pain in this trust are administered by the intravenous route using either nurse-controlled analgesia (NCA) or patient-controlled analgesia (PCA). NCA and PCA are supplemented by round-the-clock (regular) paracetamol-based analgesia with *pro re nata* (prn) tramadol, if necessary. A nurse-led pain management service is responsible for the safe provision of effective perioperative analgesia with the senior nurse accountable for regular audit and the exploration of analgesia-related adverse events.

Intravenous opioid PCA

The use of PCA has been shown to increase patient satisfaction when compared to conventional analgesia (Chumbley 2009) whilst a meta-analysis revealed higher morphine consumption but lower pain scores at 24 and 48 hours after cardiac surgery (Bainbridge *et al.* 2006). Early equipment was cumbersome and practical only for high-care clinical areas. The early 1990s saw the rapid development of disposable mechanical PCA devices using a range of delivery methods including elastomeric reservoirs and press button wristwatches. The gradual reduction in the size of electronically controlled devices encouraged the use of PCA beyond critical care areas and into the surgical wards.

PCA allows patients to manage their own analgesic intake in response to an awareness of increasing pain. After receiving an opioid loading dose to achieve the blood minimum effective analgesic concentration (usually in recovery), patients assume responsibility for their future opioid delivery by pressing a demand button to request a dose. PCA avoids the peaks and troughs associated with intramuscular analgesia, thus avoiding the need for painful, repeated injections. PCA also alleviates the need to request analgesia from nursing staff, thus facilitating immediate delivery.

Each electronic PCA device can be individually programmed to set the loading dose, bolus dose, dose duration, dose limits (e.g. over 1 or 4 hours) and whether a background infusion is required. Prescriptions vary between institutions, but intravenous morphine PCA with a 1 mg bolus and 5-minute lockout could be considered the standard. The lockout time refers to the predetermined length of time during which the device will not deliver a dose, even though a patient may make repeated requests.

PCA is associated with prescribing, dosing and administration errors (Syed *et al.* 2006; Hicks *et al.* 2008; ISMP 2008) as well as adverse events such as reactions to opioids (Hankin *et al.* 2007). The use of pre-printed prescriptions may reduce the risk of prescribing errors, but programming errors such as the incorrect inputting of the opioid concentration result in what is known as 'inverse relationships' (ISMP 2008) can still occur. If the actual concentration of opioid was programmed incorrectly as a lower concentration, e.g. if 0.1 mg/mL was programmed instead of 1 mg/mL, this would result in a tenfold bolus being delivered if a dose was requested. In an opioid-naive patient this could result in oversedation and possible respiratory depression. In addition to programming errors, demands for analgesia made by persons other than the patient can also result in respiratory depression (Hicks *et al.* 2008).

In the USA a 5-year retrospective analysis of the national voluntary MRAE database Medmarx revealed 9571 PCA-related adverse events, which represented approximately 1% of the total reported MRAEs. Incorrect dosing accounted for over 38% of errors, human factors being the main cause with nurses implicated in almost three quarters of events (Hicks *et al.* 2008).

Epidural analgesia

The delivery of local anaesthetics and opioids into the epidural space is an effective method of providing analgesia for the management of acute pain. Epidural analgesia is known to ameliorate the stress response to major abdominal surgery (Ahlers *et al.* 2008) and potentiate the effect of an amino acid infusion to reduce catabolism in patients with type 2 diabetes mellitus undergoing colonic surgery (Lugli *et al.* 2008). A review of best evidence in cardiac surgery showed that combining general anaesthesia with thoracic epidural analgesia results in shorter time to extubation and significantly better pain relief but did not reduce hospital length of stay (Ronald *et al.* 2005).

The provision of epidural analgesia is achieved by the aseptic placement of a sterile catheter into the epidural space, which is then secured to the patient's back using a dressing, which facilitates observation of the insertion site. The catheter end is connected to a sterile bacterial/particulate filter. The filter may be capped off or an infusion may be commenced. The infusion may be either patient-controlled (a combination of a background infusion with the ability for the patient to request and receive a bolus dose) or continuous nurse-controlled infusion. The infusion may contain a local anaesthetic alone or in combination with an opioid. Delivery may be achieved via the use of a syringe driver or infusion device.

Epidural analgesia is associated with potentially serious adverse effects, including nerve, dura or pleural damage at the time of catheter insertion (Royal College of Anaesthetists 2006), local anaesthetic toxicity, as well as prescribing, dosing and administration errors (as illustrated in the recent media cases).

Analgesic medicines and risk

Human factors remain a central concern in MRAEs. A number of strategies have been described to minimise MRAEs, including medication reconciliation (National Prescribing Centre 2008), the introduction of an adverse event hotline, increased reporting and feedback (NPSA 2007c), standardised infusions, tighter management of stock levels and storage (Vincent 2006) and pharmacist interventions (Liew 2008).

Nursing contribution to medicines management

Until the publication of *A Spoonful of Sugar* (Audit Commission 2001) nursing involvement in medicines management was limited – it was primarily undertaken by pharmacists. This document encouraged hospital pharmacies to engage with decision-makers to improve medicines management from selection, procurement and delivery through to prescribing and administration. In 2007 the DH published further guidance on incorporating risk management into practice (DH 2007). This document built on an earlier publication (*An Organisation with a Memory*), which had a variety of aims, including reducing serious MRAEs by 40% by the end of 2005 and highlighting the danger of intrathecal 'maladministration' (DH 2000).

New role

The development and initiation of a local medication safety initiative (MSI) group led by the lead clinician for clinical risk (a qualified anaesthetist) provided an opportunity for nurses to contribute to improving medicines management.

The MSI group membership has remained constant since inception and reflects the nature of our specialist cardiothoracic trust.

MSI group members include:

- lead clinician clinical risk (chair)
- director of pharmacy
- clinical governance and research pharmacist
- senior principal pharmacist
- senior nurse manager paediatrics
- consultant intensivist, paediatrics
- senior nurse, pain management
- senior nurse educator
- non-medical prescribing representative
- lead, clinical engineering
- consultant anaesthetist

I was initially approached to join the group as opioid medicines and their routes of delivery were seen as 'high risk' and because of my long-term interest in improving patient safety. The nurse educator who facilitates the intravenous study days which are compulsory for all nursing staff was invited, as she influenced the trust educational strategy.

Blurring of roles

Until the initiation of the MSI, medicines management was seen as the sole preserve of pharmacy. The director of pharmacy had raised the profile of the department in response to *A Spoonful of Sugar* (Audit Commission 2001), with pharmacy staff concentrating on their clinical, patient-centred roles. Nurses until this point had only been involved in medicines management with reference to severe MRAEs and the ward storage of medicines.

Prescription charts were viewed as belonging to pharmacy, with the development of those in use at the start of the MSI led by pharmacists. Analgesia prescriptions were handwritten on the reverse of the standard drug chart.

Developing the service

Improving the sensitivity of incident reporting

MRAEs prior to MSI were reported either as an adverse event through the clinical risk reporting system (known as the IR1 form) or via the local pharmacy reporting system. The IR1 system was a comprehensive A1 size triplicate form which was time-consuming to complete and was mainly used to report known adverse events or where patients experienced harm, e.g. incorrect route of administration or incorrect doses. It was not used to report 'near misses'. This generic system was used to report in hospital events of all types including falls and hospital acquired infections.

A more sensitive reporting system that could be used to collate and identify MRAEs by type (dispensing, supply, administration) and sub-type (incorrect dose, incorrect frequency, incorrect medicine) was needed if lessons were to be learnt that could positively influence practice. The clinical risk department assisted by pharmacy embarked on raising the awareness of MRAEs through a programme of education and of reporting not only actual events but near misses.

A new more sensitive electronic reporting system (Datix®) was introduced, and quarterly MRAE's reports were collated by the lead clinician for clinical risk and were distributed to the MSI members for review.

Rationale for a nurse-led analgesia programme for improving patient safety

These quarterly reports facilitated analysis of MRAEs by MSI members. Once themes were identified, MSI members were responsible for producing and initiating an action plan for each event. My specific responsibility was for all analgesia-related events and near misses.

Numerous analgesia-related themes emerged, which I classified into three main categories for ease:

(1) Oral opioids (prescribing, doses, frequency, presentations);
(2) Intravenous opioid PCA (prescribing, preparation and administration of PCA, patient observations);
(3) Epidural infusions (prescribing, preparation, presentations, administration, patient observations).

Key stakeholders

To enhance the provision of safer analgesia it was necessary to engage with specific pharmacists (director, governance, specialist pain and surgical clinical pharmacists), members of nursing and quality (director, head nurse, nurse educators, modern matrons), ward staff (sisters, charge nurses, recovery practitioners, pain link nurses) and the Department of Anaesthesia. As my trust consists of two geographically isolated hospitals, it was essential to ensure representation from both.

Influencing people to contribute to the changes

Each category of analgesia (oral, intravenous and epidural) needed a different approach and I initially set up a working party for each, although overlaps existed. I contacted staff that I thought were essential to make change happen. It was important that clinical nurses were well represented, as they were essential to the success of each initiative. At the initial meeting of each working party I presented the clinical risk data for the previous year together with any local audit or published national data. It was suggested at the very first meeting convened to review oral opioids that patients receiving PCA would be likely to receive oral opioids once the infusion has stopped and that a single working party could reduce workload and overlap.

I then sought and tested ideas for improving analgesia provision and reducing risk. An overview of function, action plans and outcomes of the two final working parties are described below.

Oral and PCA analgesia

Previous audit data from the pain service revealed that the effectiveness of oral analgesia was inadequately recorded on existing documentation and pain intensity scores were less likely to be assessed and recorded compared to patients receiving intravenous PCA or epidural analgesia. The patient's pain history was often not recorded perhaps because current documentation did not encourage nurses to ask the patient. The lack of assessment documentation has been reported elsewhere (Powell *et al.* 2009) and is likely to lead to under treatment of pain by nurses (Agency for Healthcare Policy and Research 1994). The role of the pharmacist was seen to be limited to medicines reconciliation (recorded only the prescription chart), potential interactions and ensuring that discharge medications were prescribed appropriately.

A review of the MRAEs reported to clinical risk revealed that nurses were responsible for the majority of oral and intravenous opioid errors including:

- Selecting and administering an incorrect oral opioid formulation (e.g. prolonged release OxyContin® instead of immediate release OxyNorm®);
- Making concentration errors when preparing morphine PCA bags;
- PCA device programming errors.

New documentation for oral analgesia and PCA opioids

The working party agreed to review all documentation related to oral and PCA opioids, with the aim of producing a single document that could be used from admission to discharge. I produced a number of draft documents which were reviewed and the final document which incorporated a pain history, troubleshooting guidelines and a record of assessment which was then piloted. Feedback from recovery and ward nurses was very positive with suggestions about additional information related to the frequency of observations as identified in the trust policy incorporated into the final draft design.

The final document cover (Figure 5.1) providing contact details for the pain specialist nurses, on-call anaesthetist and pain pharmacist was sent to a graphic designer before being launched. The pain assessment tool was simplified and reflected our patient population (Figure 5.2). I chose to employ a graphic designer as I wanted the document to be aesthetically pleasing, easy to use, readily identifiable and colourful. I chose a green border for this document, as this was one of the few colours not already in use for trust documents. As the document was only an assessment record and not a prescription chart, it was not necessary for ratification by the Drugs and Therapeutics Committee.

IV / PCA / Enteral Analgesia
Pain Assessment Chart

Royal Brompton & Harefield **NHS**
NHS Trust

Patient name	Consultant surgeon
Hospital number	Procedure
Date of birth	Date of surgery
Ward	Consultant anaesthetist
Known sensitivities/allergies	Weight in kg

ANALGESIA

Record of analgesia			
Analgesic		Bolus dose	
Diluent		Lockout time (mins)	
Background infusion?		Four-hour limit?	
PCA / infusion type		PCA / infusion device number	

PATIENT HISTORY

Pain history and analgesia on admission

CONTACTS

Harefield Hospital pain management service		Royal Brompton Hospital pain management service	
Pain nurse	Bleep 6144 or 6165	Pain nurse	Bleep 7037 or 7064
Pain pharmacist	Bleep 6127	Pain pharmacist	Bleep 7408
On call anaesthetist	Bleep 6102	On call anaesthetist	Bleep 1401

Figure 5.1 Cover page of IV/PCA/Enteral Pain Assessment Chart. (Reproduced with kind permission of © Royal Brompton & Harefield NHS Foundation Trust.)

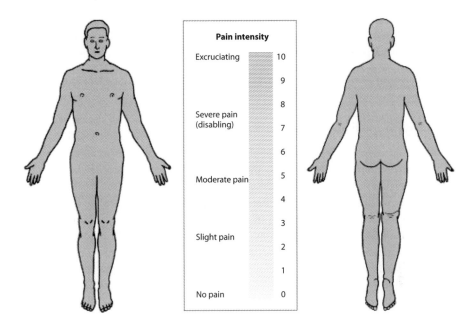

Graphic guide and descriptors based on the McGill Pain Questionnaire:

Melzack R *The McGill Pain Questionnaire: major properties and scoring methods*
Pain (1975) 1:277–299

Supplementary analogue guide:

Bourbonnais F *Pain Assessment: development of a tool for the nurse and the patient*
Journal of Advanced Nursing (1981) 6:277–282

Figure 5.2   Pain assessment tool from IV/PCA/Enteral Pain Assessment Chart. (Reproduced with kind permission of © Royal Brompton & Harefield NHS Foundation Trust.)

I ordered an initial print run of 2500 documents so that all clinical areas would have stock before the launch event. For ease of future ordering by administrative staff, I spoke with the supplies department and the trust printers for this document to be a stock item (like the standard drug chart). The cost of subsequent stock orders would be borne by the clinical area which ordered them.

Commercially prepared morphine PCA infusions

It was agreed by the director of pharmacy, governance and specialist pain pharmacists that a commercially prepared morphine bag was now appropriate in an attempt to eliminate concentration errors identified by a cluster of MRAEs. The specialist pain pharmacist and I identified three suppliers in the UK of so-called specials that would consider supplying morphine in our desired preparation of 1 mg/mL – total volume 100 mL. Of the three potential suppliers, only one could guarantee that the final concentration of morphine in the bag would be 1 mg/mL as the other two did not produce bags from scratch but added morphine concentrate into sodium chloride 0.9% 100 mL bags which already contained in excess of 100 mL, as providing an overfill ($\approx$5%) is standard practice.

Once the supplier was agreed the projected number of bags required per annum was calculated by contacting the supplies department to determine the number of PCA administration sets ordered per annum and comparing this against the number of morphine sulphate 30 mg for injection ampoules ordered by pharmacy each year. The higher the projected number, the lower the unit price. The price quoted by the manufacturer was just over £7 per unit, which was disputed by the director of pharmacy as too expensive but I was able to demonstrate that the nursing time coupled with the cost of disposables needed to make a bag from scratch in recovery (where I had timed how long it took to make up a bag) where comparable.

Storage of the new minibags was not an issue in the clinical areas as new controlled drugs (CD) cupboards had recently been installed. Stock levels of the new minibags were agreed with the lead nurse for each clinical area and ward pharmacist. Stock of morphine sulphate 30 mg for injection was removed from all clinical areas as it was no longer required. This would further reduce the chances of an inappropriate concentration of morphine being selected for other purposes.

Enhancing PCA infusion safety

Once the new documentation had been approved and implemented, clinical engineering was approached to assist in streamlining the infusion devices used for PCA delivery. Although the trust had merged in 1997, the infusion devices used for PCA in the two hospitals were different, although an identical device (yellow GemStar®, Hospira) had recently been introduced for epidural analgesia. It was agreed that the trust should be aiming to have a fleet of identical pumps as this would have beneficial effects upon training, disposable purchase prices and maintenance.

Negotiations were extended as funding ($\sim$50K) needed to be sought to facilitate this. The introduction of a GemStar® device with blue fascia to make it recognisably different from the yellow epidural device occurred approximately 8 months after agreement was reached that device was necessary. The launch was preceded by an intensive 8-week competency-based training programme which was undertaken by specialist pain nurses aided by link nurses in each clinical area. The PCA devices were programmed to ensure that patients received only a continuous infusion (nurse-controlled) of opioid or a bolus only (patient-controlled) programme.

The PCA policy and separate guideline were updated and ratified by the Drugs and Therapeutics Committee to reflect the single device now used for PCA infusions. The guideline was necessary as although PCA primarily used morphine sulphate, intravenous Fentanyl and oxycodone are also used in patients unsuitable for morphine because of sensitivity, allergy or altered renal function. To ensure that PCA infusions were distinct from intravenous and epidural infusions, a green 'PCA' sticker was applied on the administration set close to the pump and also near the patient's peripheral cannula. These green PCA stickers coordinated with the green assessment document.

Epidural analgesia

Although similar in structure and function to the multidisciplinary working party for oral and PCA analgesia, the aims of the epidural working party was complicated by the publication of 'Safer practice with epidural injections and infusions' (NPSA 2007b). This document made six recommendations for action for the NHS and independent sector in England and Wales:

(1) Clearly label infusion bags and syringes for 'Epidural Use Only' with the judicious use of colour;
(2) Minimise the likelihood of confusion between different types and strengths of epidural injections and infusions:
    (a) Rationalise the range of infusates and undertake an annual audit;
    (b) Maximise the use of ready-to-use infusions;
(3) Store epidurals in separate cupboards;
(4) Clearly label administration sets and catheters;
(5) Use infusion devices that are easily distinguishable from other types of infusions;
(6) Ensure all staff have received adequate training and completed competencies.

Although I assumed leadership of the epidural working party, I was now responsible for the trust response to the NPSA about progress in achieving their recommendations.

Updated documentation for epidural analgesia

The epidural prescription had historically been handwritten on a separate red A4 piece of paper with an adhesive strip. Once completed the prescription was adhered to the intravenous section of the drug chart. The prescription was reviewed and represcribed daily with bolus doses, if required, prescribed on the same document. The working group agreed that all epidural documentation should be combined, and to achieve this, a combined prescription, troubleshooting and assessment document would be the ideal.

To have a single document with a limited choice of infusates from a pre-printed list, consensus from the prescribing anaesthetists was essential. The range of infusates employed in the trust needed to reflect our use of predominantly thoracic epidural analgesia and employ the 'safer' local anaesthetics that were on the market.

Patient education

In addition to the development of a pre-operative patient information booklet about the risks and benefits of regional analgesia, the need for a patient educational leaflet to highlight potentially serious sequelae related to epidural catheter removal, i.e. epidural haematoma and abscess formation, was discussed by the working party. The pain management service (PMS) had published an internal guideline for clinical staff that detailed low-molecular-weight heparin, thromboprophylaxis and the timings of epidural catheter insertion and removal from patients should be managed. However, in response to an increased public awareness of epidural abscess formation after recent media attention, it was agreed to produce a patient information leaflet which outlined the signs and symptoms of haematoma and abscess formation and the importance of seeking early medical advice. After wide consultation with clinical staff a draft document was piloted with five patients in each clinical area. Formal evaluation of the content, layout and suitability was undertaken and use of this document is now standard practice.

Working with industry

At this time a variety of infusates were employed, reflecting individual prescriber's standard practices. The local anaesthetic most frequently prescribed was bupivacaine 0.1% (although 0.15% was used for approximately 10% of infusions) either as a plain infusion or in combination with Fentanyl (range from 2 to 5 mcg/mL). Commercially prepared bupivacaine 0.1% with Fentanyl 2 mcg/mL (250 mL volume) was on formulary and was available in all clinical areas. Fentanyl was added to commercially prepared plain bupivacaine 0.1% bags (100 mL volume) by nurses in the clinical areas if a higher Fentanyl concentration (i.e. >2 mcg/mL) was desired. This was not ideal as dosing errors had occurred and there were infection control and prevention issues associated with adding an additive to a bag which would then be punctured again by the administration set spike.

I undertook a postal survey of all consultant anaesthetists in the trust asking what their ideal local anaesthetic and local anaesthetic in combination with Fentanyl presentations would be. The results of the survey indicated that we should limit the infusates to two presentations: a plain local anaesthetic and a local anaesthetic in combination with Fentanyl, although the desired Fentanyl concentrations ranged from 2 to 5 mcg/mL with no clear majority. There was consensus that if a 'safer' local anaesthetic such as levobupivacaine was available then this should be in use.

Simultaneously I approached industry to determine what solutions were available currently and what the manufacturing possibilities were. Only one 'specials' manufacturer, Fresenius Kabi, who produced our current bupivacaine infusions, was interested in the possibility of working with a trust to develop a new product. The manager responsible for 'specials' asked if she could come and meet with the team and spend some time with the PMS to see how we used products in practice and to learn more about the practical issues associated with them.

It was important that industry understood the needs of the clinician and that we clinicians understood the practical and commercial realities. The meeting between industry and the working party went very smoothly. It was explained to us that if we wished to have levobupivacaine (manufactured and marketed exclusively by Abbott Laboratories as Chirocaine®) in combination with Fentanyl produced as a 'special', this combination was unlicensed and would require stability testing that would take over 12 months.

I had produced a list of desirable characteristics of the final product, which included the volume of the preparation and the need for distinct labelling and overlabelling. The group agreed that a volume of 500 mL would be ideal as a single bag would provide sufficient volume for the majority of post-operative patients; thus the bag would not need changing for the 'average' patient. This would reduce the risk of administration errors and the possibility of contamination from an infection prevention perspective. After reviewing the literature and in response to the survey of anaesthetist's current practices, it was decided by me and the two hospital lead anaesthetists for acute pain that we would like to have levobupivacaine 0.125% and Fentanyl 4 mcg/mL in a 500-mL bag.

Spending time in the clinical environment raised the awareness of the industry representative of the need to reduce the potential safety concerns associated with this 'high-risk' route and that the new package needed to be distinctly visually different from the plain local anaesthetic infusion.

Over the next month I undertook an electronic survey of my colleagues in the London region to gauge interest in a levobupivacaine–Fentanyl preparation. This sample was convenient as the RCN London Pain Forum meets regularly and has an excellent electronic format for asking pain-related queries. A number of trusts expressed interest. I had also been in contact with Abbott Laboratories and had determined that they had marketing authorisation and were preparing to launch levobupivacaine 0.125% 200-mL bags licensed for epidural use.

Once the stability testing had been completed by Fresenius Kabi, I was approached by them to review the bag labelling and overlabelling. In response to my comments, they amended the printing on the actual bag so that 'For Epidural Use Only' was boxed yellow text (no longer black) and agreed that the overwrapper should be distinctly different from intravenous infusions. I was asked to review a unique striped wrapper and I agreed that it would make this infusate easy to distinguish from one for administration by other routes, e.g. intravenous. Of note is that a recent document from the NPSA patient safety division now recommends the use of colour on bags, although the example given in this document illustrates the use of bupivacaine and not the 'safer' local anaesthetic levobupivacaine (NPSA 2008).

Drugs and Therapeutics Committee approval

Chaired by a practising medically qualified clinician, our trust committee approves all new medicines and new formulations together with all medicine-related documentation (policies, guidelines, prescriptions, etc.). Although standard practice in all health care institutions in the UK, this committee is often viewed as a major challenge when expanding a team's formulary or developing a service. In addition to

providing a critical appraisal of the evidence together with any projected cost implications weeks in advance of the meeting, a presentation is required that explains what
the benefits are to the service and to the patient. The publication of the NPSA (2007b)
supported our changes in infusates, although the anticipated expenditure in the budget
was a 10% increase. The committee supported the proposal and tasked the specialist
pharmacist for surgery and pain to deal with supply issues.

The final yellow comprehensive epidural prescription (Figure 5.3) and assessment
document produced by the graphic designer was broadly welcomed by the committee
even though the director of pharmacy did not fully support the introduction of an
additional prescription document. In response to the committee's approval of the
infusates and the updated documentation, I arranged for a print run of the document
to be ready for the launch of the new infusates in 2 months' time. This would allow
Fresenius Kabi sufficient time to produce a batch and to publicise the launch of the
new products within the trust.

Safer epidural storage and administration

Until the publication of a draft version in July 2006 of the final epidural alert (NPSA
2007b) the storage of epidural infusates had not been considered a priority by pharmacy, the PMS or ward nursing staff. It was agreed that the introduction of the
morphine bags for PCA use reduced space in the CD cupboard, but the alert required
separate storage of epidural infusates.

Visits to all clinical areas were undertaken with the ward sister and pharmacist
responsible for each area to identify risks and also to suggest sensible alternatives.
Pharmacy suggested that the plain 200-mL local anaesthetic bags could be stored in a
labelled box in the oral medicines cabinet in each clinical area. It was agreed that the
morphine PCA bags could safely remain in the current CD cabinet alongside oral, injectable and transdermal opioids, whilst the opioid containing epidural bags should be
stored in a separate clearly labelled cupboard that conformed to regulations for CDs.
This meant that each clinical area would need to order an additional cabinet, the dimensions of which was based upon agreed stock levels and available suitable wall space.
CD cabinets in the UK are made to order and there is a 6–10-week waiting time from order to delivery. As I was responsible for the trust response to the alert, I was also tasked
by the director of pharmacy to supervise the mounting of all cabinets by the carpenter.

Challenges in implementing the changes in practice

Business strategy

Determining the financial impact of any new intervention is essential. It requires
an accurate assessment of projected costs and savings and should provide future
projections. Budget holders and business managers must be engaged as they can
facilitate pump priming and assist in the reallocation of funds from one cost stream to
another. A business strategy was developed for both the PCA and epidural projects.

Epidural Analgesia Prescription

Royal Brompton & Harefield **NHS**
NHS Trust

EPIDURAL

Patient name

Hospital number

Date of birth

Ward

Known sensitivities/allergies

Consultant surgeon

Procedure

Date of surgery

Consultant anaesthetist

Weight in kg | Pharmacy use only

Inserted at _____ to _____ depth _____ cm

EPIDURAL SOLUTION

Date	Solution	Volume	Rate range	Doctor's signature
	Levobupivacaine 0.125% + fentanyl 4mcg/ml in sodium chloride 0.9%			
	Levobupivacaine 0.125% in sodium chloride 0.9%			
	Levobupivacaine 0.125% + fentanyl _____ mcg/ml in sodium chloride 0.9%			
	Levobupivacaine 0.125% + diamorphine _____ mg in sodium chloride 0.9%			

INFUSIONS

Date	Time	Infusion type	Volume	Initial (nurse 1)	Initial (nurse 2)

BOLUS/TOP-UPS

Date	Time	Drug(s)	Volume	Anaesthetist's signature

RB100

Figure 5.3 Cover page of Epidural Prescription Chart. (Reproduced with kind permission of © Royal Brompton & Harefield NHS Foundation Trust.)

I considered it necessary to produce separate plans as different stakeholders were involved and the cost of making epidural practice safer was considerable.

The PCA business case included but was not limited to:

- An overview of PCA-related MRAEs and the PCA project from a patient safety and human factors perspective together with detailed information from clinical engineering;
- Projected cost of morphine minibags per annum;
- Projected cost of purchase of the fleet of GemStar$^{®}$ infusion devices and disposables (which included a training package provided by industry);
- Cost of graphic designer to produce final assessment document;
- Print cost of assessment document and PCA stickers per annum;
- Reduction in morphine sulphate ampoule use and dispensing/supply costs;
- Reduction in nursing hours for infusion preparation;
- Reduction in MRAEs related to PCA with subsequent reduction in investigator hours.

The epidural business case included, but was not limited, to:

- An overview of NPSA recommendations, epidural-related MRAEs and the objectives of the project working group;
- Projected costs of levobupivacaine and levobupivacaine in combination with Fentanyl minibags (and cost savings from eliminating bupivacaine solutions);
- Projected cost of GemStar$^{®}$ fleet expansion;
- Cost of each clinical area purchasing a new CD regulations compliant cupboard for CD-containing minibags;
- Cost of graphic designer to produce the epidural prescription and comprehensive assessment document;
- Print cost of the epidural document and stickers per annum;
- Reduction in MRAEs related to epidurals with subsequent reduction in investigator hours.

Multidisciplinary working

One of the major challenges for me as a specialist nurse was to be seen by some of the disciplines as the clinical lead for the PMS rather than that post being held by the traditional anaesthetist. As the work streams of the collaborative working parties intensified, attitudes changed. Although enthusiasm fluctuated, this positive shift in attitude advanced as each member gained a more thorough understanding of each other's roles. The clinical nurses of the pain service gained through collaborative working. They developed their knowledge of change and project management plus the need for engagement at all levels, which is essential for success.

The epidural project was a runner-up for the annual Mallabar Award given by the Foundation of Nursing Studies and was the subject of a number of interdisciplinary published papers and conference presentations (Cox *et al.* 2007; Cox & Scott 2008; Liew 2008). The comprehensive epidural prescription chart and the patient information leaflet (haematomas and abscesses) have subsequently been adapted for use in other trusts in England and Northern Ireland.

The support of the MSI was invaluable as were the contributions from the nurse educator (for the development of the multidisciplinary competencies), the specialist pharmacists and the hospital leads for risk management. The assistance from industry was a result of collaborative working and an understanding of the needs of industry balanced by the needs of the end user (the clinician). The increasing awareness of the patient safety agenda through the NPSA and the Patient Safety First campaign has helped drive the success of these two projects, although work continues, for instance, on enhancing the safety of neuraxial delivery systems and medicines packaging and labelling.

Ongoing evaluation and audit

Clinical audit

For projects of this nature, quantitative data were considered to be of most use. Audit data from the quarterly MRAEs reports and other snapshot audits related to practice issues continue to be utilised to enhance practice. For example, in critical care the MRAEs data are fed back to all staff on team days by a presentation from a pain nurse specialist. This enables clinical nurses to explore individual events and develop agreed action plans to minimise the potential for recurrence. In addition, it raises the profile of the work of the MSI, the need to report MRAEs and near misses and reinforces that reporters of adverse events can do so within a 'blame-free' culture.

Specific audits have been undertaken in clinical areas that had been considered 'high risk'. For example, critical care has seen a reduction in the number and severity of epidural analgesia events from seven reports in 2001 (43% amber rating indicating significant patient impact using NPSA criteria), six reports in 2006 to three reports in 2007 (no patients experiencing any significant harm) (Cox *et al.* 2008).

Other smaller snapshot audits have been undertaken to assess the effectiveness of the education programme, competency completion and trust policy adherence. A snapshot audit was undertaken, with data collection repeated daily over a 5-day period, with all patients in the trust receiving epidural or PCA analgesia were included. Data collected included that the infusion device was appropriate and programmed correctly, that administration sets were correct and labelled according to policy and that nurses had completed the appropriate competencies and had attended the necessary study days. The results from this audit informed the education programme and necessitated meetings with clinical educators and the Learning & Development Department to ensure that competencies were completed and that additional classroom time was required to facilitate study days.

Service feedback from staff

Evaluation data from the epidural study day were overwhelmingly positive, but it was suggested that the pain study day could be held over 2 days to allow staff greater exposure to practical issues such as infusion device training as recommended by Cousins (2009).

A multidisciplinary focus group was convened to explore the service needs of trust users and potential areas that could be improved. This was undertaken approximately 12 months after the introduction of the commercially prepared PCA and epidural infusates. Staff were divided into small groups and asked to identify the five key strengths and five weaknesses of the PMS. Apart from the desire by ward nurses to have a 7-day service from the PMS (which currently has weekend and out of hours cover provided by critical care outreach and the post-fellowship anaesthetist on call), the themes were common to all groups and were overwhelmingly positive. It was encouraging for the PMS team to learn from prescribers, pharmacists and nurses that the new documentation, infusion devices and infusates were now seen as essential tools.

Comments recorded during the discussion after the group work included:

[N]ot needing to change the epidural bag even after the drains are removed is brilliant. (Ward nurse)

I feel quite confident to re-programme the PCA pump if I need to change a bag. I also like to see the patient's pain history on the front of the chart. . . makes it easier. (Ward nurse)

I really like the yellow epidural chart. It co-ordinates with the pump and giving set. (Recovery practitioner)

I can see from the end of the bed if the patient has a PCA or an epidural because I can see the stickers. I like that. It makes bedside handover easier. (Ward nurse)

[B]eing able to review previous solution changes and prescribe boluses on the front of the epidural chart reduces the time it takes to top-up the patient. (Anaesthetist)

Justifying the advanced nursing contribution

My role as the senior nurse (and lead clinician) responsible for cross trust analgesia provision meant that I was in a unique position. Working at an advanced level, responsible for local service provision, I was involved at a regional and national level in issues related to perioperative pain. I was experienced at interpreting, adapting and disseminating British, European and international evidence, policies and guidelines for local use. My managerial and budgetary experience enabled me to write compelling business plans to support all of these initiatives and to expand the nursing establishment. To raise the profile of the service, the MSI and medication safety in general, I regularly contributed to local publications, the national nursing press and undertook conference presentations. This enabled me to raise not only the profile of specialist nursing within the trust but provided evidence of dissemination to management to encourage ongoing financial support to the PMS.

Local evidence for the need to change resulted from the trust analgesia-related MRAEs, which were supported by recommendations from national bodies such as the NPSA. To gain support to enhance analgesia safety I needed to be able to make staff aware of the current levels of risk, adverse event reports and near misses. I utilised the media attention on fatalities associated with inadvertent intravenous local anaesthetic administration and the reports of abscesses to drive this project. Support from the multidisciplinary pain team (nurses, anaesthetists, pharmacists, physiotherapists and psychologists) was fundamental to the evolution and success of the project.

Conclusions

Providing safer post-operative analgesia using high-risk routes has required a thorough review of all practices and utilising the skills of the wider team. Improving medication safety requires a multidisciplinary approach that needs to encompass education, training and competency-based assessment. To reduce MRAEs, the presentation, ordering, prescribing, supply, storage and administration must be evaluated and enhanced. The nursing contribution to this medium-term project in a specialist cardiothoracic trust has resulted in significant benefits to staff and patients.

The intravenous route for PCA is convenient as absorption of the analgesic is not dependent upon gastric emptying as a result of anaesthesia and the patient is placed in charge of their own analgesia delivery. This route is not without risk as evidenced by local MRAEs reports and repeated errors with preparation and administration of opioid PCA. These issues are universal and have been identified in the published literature (Syed *et al.* 2006; Hicks *et al.* 2008; ISMP 2008). The standardisation of PCA prescriptions, the introduction of a commercially prepared infusate and a single infusion device with imbedded safety parameters have reduced the incidence of PCA-related MRAEs. The development and introduction of specific documentation has improved the quality and frequency of pain assessment and highlighted the importance of a patient's pain history. The colour coordination of the green PCA documentation and identifying green stickers has contributed to medication safety.

The development of the MSI led by a champion of risk reduction meant that I had regular exposure to an interdisciplinary team with shared interests but diverse knowledge, skills and experience. The enthusiasm and support of the MSI encouraged me to gain the support of the necessary individuals and teams to drive the changes in practice that I was able to effect.

I hope this project will encourage others to review MRAEs and develop an action plan with input and cooperation from the multidisciplinary team, despite the challenges associated with the Drugs and Therapeutics Committee. My action plan was diverse from developing patient educational materials in response to media attention through to gaining managerial support to provide the funds to expand the nursing contribution and rationalise infusion devices. The benefits of this project extend beyond analgesia provision. The profile and value of the pain service have been raised as has the need for greater care to ensure safer prescribing, supply, storage and administration of all medicines.

References

Agency for Healthcare Policy and Research, 1994. *Management of Cancer Pain: Clinical Practice Guidelines*, no.9 (ACPHR publication 94-0592). Rockville: Department of Health and Human Services.

Ahlers, O., Nachtigall, I., Lenze, J., Goldman, A., Schulte, E., Höhne, C., Fritz, G., Keh, D., 2008. Intraoperative thoracic epidural analgesia attenuates the stress-induced immunosuppression in patients undergoing major abdominal surgery. *British Journal of Anaesthesia*, 101(6), 781–787.

Astra Zeneca, 2005. Marcain polyamp 0.25% and 0.5% special product characteristics. Available at http://emc.medicines.org.uk/medicine/9367/SPC/Marcain+Polyamp+Steripack+0.25%25+and+0.5%25/ [accessed 22 February 2009].

Audit Commission, 2001. *A Spoonful of Sugar; Medicines Management in NHS Hospitals*. London: NPSA. Available at http://www.audit-commission.gov.uk/reports/AC-REPORT.asp?CatID=&ProdID=E83C8921-6CEA-4b2c-83E7-F80954A80F85 [accessed 23 February 2009].

Bainbridge, D., Martin, J.E., Cheng, D.C., 2006. Patient-controlled versus nurse-controlled analgesia after cardiac surgery – a meta-analysis. *Canadian Journal of Anaesthesia*, 53(5), 492–499.

Chumbley, G., 2009. Patient controlled analgesia. In Cox, F. (ed.), *Perioperative Pain Management*. p 161–185. Oxford: Wiley-Blackwell.

Cousins, A., 2009. Education. In Cox, F. (ed.), *Perioperative Pain Management*. p 294–309. Oxford: Wiley-Blackwell.

Cox, F., Cousins, A., Smith, A., Marwick, C., Gullberg, C., 2007. Acute pain management after major thoracic surgery. *Nursing Times*, 103(23), 30–31.

Cox, F., Scott, K., 2008. Improving epidural safety through new documentation. *Nursing Times*, 104(12), 26–27.

Cox, F.J., Smith, A., Mitchell, J.B., Farrimond, J.G., 2008. Reducing risk with thoracic epidural analgesia in critical care. *Poster presented at ESICM*. Lisbon.

Department of Health, 2000. *An Organization with a Memory*. London: DH. Available at http://www.dh.gov.uk/en/Publicationsandstatistics/Publications/PublicationsPolicyAndGuidance/DH_4065083 [accessed 13 March 2009].

Department of Health, 2007. Building a safer NHS for patients: implementing an organization with a memory. Available at http://www.dh.gov.uk/en/Publicationsandstatistics/Publications/PublicationsPolicyAndGuidance/Browsable/DH_4097460 [accessed 13 March 2009].

Department of Health, 2008. *Heath Service Circular 2008/001 Updated National Guidance on the Safe Administration of Intrathecal Chemotherapy*. London: DH. Available at http://www.dh.gov.uk/en/Publicationsandstatistics/Lettersandcirculars/Healthservicecirculars/DH_086870 [accessed 23 February 2009].

Department of Health, 2009. Hospital episode data. Available at www.hesonline.nhs.uk [accessed 22 February 2009].

Hankin, C.S., Schein, J., Clark, J.A., Panchal, S., 2007. Adverse events involving patient-controlled analgesia. *American Journal of Health-System Pharmacy*, 64(14), 1492–1499.

Hicks, R.W., Sikirica, V., Nwelson, W., Schein, J.R., Cousins, D.D., 2008. Medication errors involving patient-controlled analgesia. *American Journal of Health-System Pharmacy*, 65(5), 429–440.

Institute for Safe Medication Practices, 2008. *Misprogramming PCA Concentration Leads to Dosing Errors*. Horsham PA: ISMP. Available at http://www.ismp.org/Newsletters/acutecare/articles/20080828.asp [accessed 06 March 2009].

Liew, J., 2008. A pilot study of pharmacy led patient safety contributions in a tertiary centre. *Poster Presented at the Patient Safety Congress*. London.

Lugli, A.K., Donatelli, F., Schricker, T., Wykes, L., Carli, F., 2008. Epidural analgesia enhances the postoperative anabolic effect of amino acids in diabetes mellitus type 2 patients undergoing colon surgery. *Anesthesiology*, 108(6), 1093–1099.

National Patient Safety Agency, 2007a. Patient safety alert 20. Promoting safer use of injectable medicines. Available at www.npsa.nhs.uk [accessed 06 March 2009].

National Patient Safety Agency, 2007b. Patient safety alert 21. Safer practice with epidural injections and infusions. Available at www.npsa.nhs.uk [accessed 06 March 2009].

National Patient Safety Agency, 2007c. *Safety in Doses: Medication Safety Incidents in the NHS*. London: NPSA. Available at http://www.npsa.nhs.uk/nrls/alerts-and-directives/directives-guidance/safety-in-doses/ [accessed 14 March 2009].

National Patient Safety Agency, 2008. *Design for Patient Safety: A Guide to Labelling and Packaging of Injectable Medicines*. London: NPSA.

National Prescribing Centre, 2008. Medicines reconciliation. Available at http://www.npci.org.uk/medicines_management/safety/reconcil/library/5mg_reconconciliation.php [accessed 12 March 2009].

Powell, A.E., Davies, H.T.O., Bannister, J., Macrae, W.A., 2009. Understanding the challenges of services changes – learning from acute pain services in the UK. *Journal of the Royal Society of Medicine*, 102, 62–68.

Ronald, A., Abdulaziz, K.A., Day, T.G., Scott, M., 2005. In patients undergoing cardiac surgery, thoracic epidural analgesia combined with general anaesthesia results in faster recovery and fewer complications but does not affect length of hospital stay. *Interactive Cardiovascular and Thoracic Surgery*, 5(3), 207–216.

Royal College of Anaesthetists, 2006. *Risks Associated with Your Anaesthetic. Section 11. Nerve Damage Associated with a Spinal or Epidural Injection*. London: RCoA. Available at http://www.rcoa.ac.uk/docs/nerve-spinal.pdf [accessed 11 March 2009].

Royston, D., Cox, F., 2003. Anaesthesia: the patient's point of view. *The Lancet*, 362, 1648–1658.

Syed, S., Paul, J.E., Hueftlein, M., Kampf, M., Mclean, R.F., 2006. Morphine overdose from error propagation on an acute pain service. *Canadian Journal of Anesthesia*, 53(6), 586–590.

Timesonline, 2003. Doctor admits fatal blunder over cancer boy (23 September 2003). Available at http://www.timesonline.co.uk/tol/news/uk/article1161979.ece [accessed 24 February 2009].

Timesonline, 2008a. Lesley Ash gets £5 m payout from hospital where she caught infection (17 January 2008). Available at www.timesonline.co.uk/tol/life_and_style/health/article3201003.ece [accessed 23 February 2009].

Timesonline, 2008b. Mayra Cabrera unlawfully killed by 'epidural blunder' in hospital (5 February 2008). Available at www.timesonline.co.uk/tol/life_and_style/health/article3314183.ece [accessed 23 February 2009].

Vincent, C., 2006. *Patient Safety*. London: Churchill Livingstone, Elsevier.

Internet resources

The Institute for Safe Medication Practices: www.ismp.org.

National Patient Safety Agency: www.npsa.nhs.uk.

National Prescribing Centre: www.npci.org.uk.

Patient Safety First Campaign: www.patientsafetyfirst.nhs.uk.

Royal College of Anaesthetists: www.rcoa.ac.uk.

Chapter 6
Developing an acupuncture service for chronic pain

Ruth H. Heafield, Christine M. Haigh, Christine M. Barnes and Elaine Beddingham

Introduction

The provision of pain management to those with chronic pain is not as simple as finding the individual analgesic agent or technique. The person in pain will almost certainly have other existing comorbidities and receiving a multiplicity of other treatments, prescribed medications and specialist interventions over often many years. During such varied treatment exposure over such a long time period patients have a high probability of experiencing ineffective treatments or unbearable side effects, which can lead to a reduction in their faith of orthodox medicine. Often those with chronic conditions such as pain will then seek the less orthodox approaches such as Traditional Chinese Medicine (Thomas *et al.* 2001). The problem with accessing such treatments is that there is limited provision of acupuncture within the NHS, and patients often opt to access private acupuncturists where there may not be the requirement for regulation. Registration of complementary therapists is still under debate with ministers calling for statutory regulation of such practitioners to ensure safety. The most recent report from the Department of Health (DH) Steering Group on the statutory regulation of practitioners (DH Steering Group 2008) certainly supports regulation as being in the public interest; however, this has yet to be implemented. Despite the increase in public interest and demand, many NHS trusts find themselves struggling to provide such therapies within the tight monetary constraints of the NHS particularly as complementary therapies and specifically acupuncture is seen as an 'overhead' to existing services and therefore is not paid for as a separate entity through the national tariff. This means that the funding to develop any new acupuncture services will have to be carefully considered alongside current funding streams and service pressures. This groundwork is imperative to any acupuncture service development.

The authors have over 30 years' experience between them of the development of acupuncture services within the current NHS. The aim of this chapter is to bring together their expertise and experience, through personal consultations, to provide a body of knowledge for those considering developing an acupuncture service for pain management. The advanced nurse practitioner has a key role to play to not only affect practice in their own area but also influence that of others. The chapter identifies the three key areas for consideration when developing an acupuncture service. In the first section we consider the potential size, referral systems and pathways for the service and patient journey. This provides the rationale for setting up such a service and how a service might be developed. An important part of the service development strategy is how will staff develop and maintain their competence regarding the practice of acupuncture. This is discussed separately in the following section. Finally, we consider the clinical governance issues surrounding the safety and quality of the service.

Rationale for setting up an acupuncture clinic for pain management

This section considers the process of referrals, the clinical considerations for the service and the development of treatment pathways.

Referrals

Acupuncture is available on referral from about one third of primary care trusts in the UK, usually carried out in NHS pain clinics (Drugs & Therapeutics Bulletin 2007). A number of general practitioners, nurses and physiotherapists in the community are now also providing acupuncture themselves in an attempt to provide this treatment earlier in the patients' pain management. Acupuncture is used by an estimated 2% of adults in the UK each year, with less than 10% of provision through the NHS (Thomas *et al.* 2006). Patients may be referred for acupuncture by other specialities within an acute trust, for example orthopaedic surgeons or extended scope physiotherapists.

A key consideration for those setting up acupuncture services, with regard to access to services, is where will the majority of referral come from. Will the service be suitably positioned to provide for those patients and the referrers requirements?

Generally, patients are assessed by a multiprofessional team to ascertain that acupuncture is an appropriate treatment for the type of chronic pain that is being experienced. Studies suggest that acupuncture may help a variety of pain symptoms, leading to a reduction in analgesic requirements and improvement in mobility (Filshie & Hester 2006). Acupuncture is often provided from a nurse (or physio)-led clinics where the nurse makes an assessment of the pain and decides upon point selection (the point where the needle is to be inserted), number of needles and length of time for those needles to remain in place. A discussion of the risks and benefits allows the patient to provide informed verbal consent and be treated with acupuncture (see also subsection 'Clinical governance'). The length of consultation needs to take into account the time required to provide this information and allow discussion of the potential risks and benefits.

The general approach of NHS clinics, in the UK, for chronic pain management is to provide the patient with a treatment once a week for between 4 and 6 weeks in total, followed by review and assessment. Successful treatment can be measured by continued relief of symptoms or reduction of pain combined with enhanced quality-of-life measures such as a better sleep pattern and increased function.

What constitutes an optimal course of treatment is not known, as the benefits fade over time although benefits can be reported up to 6 months after treatment for some patients. If patients do not respond after 12-weekly sessions, it is unlikely that they will respond to acupuncture and other treatment options should be considered and discussed (Filshie & Hester 2006).

A study by Thomas *et al.* (2006) demonstrated weak evidence had been found of the effect of acupuncture on non-specific back pain at 12 months with stronger evidence of small benefit at 24 months. Acupuncture is generally not seen as a cure for pain, particularly in the chronically ill, and the service has a potential to expand beyond its resources if consideration of repeat treatment times and ratios are not calculated into the service development plan. This demonstrates that it may be difficult to decide on optimal acupuncture treatment as many variables exist.

Clinical considerations

There are several important clinical considerations when setting up an acupuncture clinic. These include patient selection, contraindications (absolute and relative), potential side effects and consideration of children and those pregnant. The impact the service may have on others is considered. It is also important to identify which types of pain are potentially amenable to acupuncture. Finally, treatment pathways are described and the different types of acupuncture courses generally available.

Patient selection

A decision has to be made whether acupuncture is the suitable treatment for any given patient. Many patients may wish to try acupuncture as the media can portray it as 'a natural, alternative therapy with no potential harmful side effects'. This is not the case; a careful assessment of the potential risks versus benefits must be undertaken and discussed with the patient prior to treatment. The main ones are outlined below.

Contraindications
Absolute

- Pregnancy – uterine contractions are stimulated by using acupuncture points. Specific points are treated by midwives to induce labour and turn babies who are in the breech position. Tsuei *et al.* (1977) suggests 'any patient who may be pregnant at the time of acupuncture may be at risk of miscarriage'. Because of these risks and any potential litigation process, the lower abdomen and lumbosacral region should not be needled during the first 3 months of pregnancy (Norris 2001). After this period it is down to the local governance committees to debate the more political issues.
- Fujiwara *et al.* (1980, cited in Norris 2004) states 'patients with demand pacemakers are an absolute contraindication for electro acupuncture' (a small current is passed through the metal needles similar to transcutaneous electrical nerve stimulation [TENS]). Electroacupuncture has been demonstrated to interfere with a demand pacemaker.
- Patient refusal – an obvious contraindication.

- Metal sensitivity or allergy – an anaphylactic response may occur and require emergency resuscitation procedures. Careful needle selection and patient questioning can prevent this.
- Needle phobia – patients may require use of acupressure as needling is inappropriate. Acupressure is the stimulation of acupuncture points using the fingers and hands instead of needles (Norris 2001).

Relative

- Diabetic patients require caution as skin sensation and peripheral circulation may be altered, leading to potential skin damage with acupuncture needles, especially using the hands or feet (Norris 2001). In traditional Chinese acupuncture an extra point exists to treat diabetes; this has been demonstrated during western investigations. Specifically that acupuncture may alter blood sugar levels and patients should be warned to monitor their hypoglycaemic status (Hopwood *et al.* 1997).
- Recent seizures/epileptic fits – this is debated; however, generally acupuncture is avoided if patients have had a fit in the last 3 months (Norris 2001). The use of the fewest number of needles should be used to obtain a therapeutic response to prevent overstimulation.
- Patients with haemophilia or other bleeding disorders – who may be at risk of further bleeding from the acupuncture sites and areas treated due to their clotting dysfunction.
- Infections or broken skin over potential site for needling – risk of introducing infection through the normal skin barrier.
- Neutropenic patients – due to the increased risk of infection/sepsis.
- Valvular heart disease – due to a risk of sub-acute bacterial endocarditis developing after needling (Filshie & Hester 2006).

Potential side effects

There is an assortment of possible side effects to acupuncture with varying level of potential harm. The course of events after an initial acupuncture treatment is always unpredictable (Campbell 1998). Although relatively minor or rare side effects must be discussed, the main ones for consideration are outlined below:

- Temporary increase in pain – some patients will report worsened pain after each treatment, which may continue for 1–2 days. Patients require information about taking simple analgesia as appropriate. This increase in pain does not usually last long and may be due to over vigorous treatment. Some schools of thought see increased pain as a positive indicator that there will be a therapeutic response (Campbell 1998). Generally a reduction of the number of needles used will lessen the intensity of the pain.
- Pneumothorax – this should be avoided by good anatomical knowledge, a high degree of caution in the needling of points on the thorax and in the anterior and posterior triangles of the neck with particular attention to the depth and direction of needle insertion. Treating areas around the intercostals spaces, paraspinal areas and

supraclavicular regions have resulted in damage to the pleura, leading to bilateral or unilateral pneumothorax. This is a key area of the practitioner training.

- Cardiac tamponade – care and prevention must also be taken not to needle deeply over the sternum as 8% of the population have foramen sternale where the central portion of the sternum fails to ossify during adolescence. A membrane covers the sternum instead of bone and if needled at point CV17, it could result in trauma to the pericardium and cardiac tamponade (Norris 2001).
- Bruising at the needle site – withdrawal of the needle may be followed by slight bleeding easily stopped by applying light pressure. A bruise or haematoma may appear. Patients just need to be warned routinely about this potential problem to prevent distress.
- Sickness/nausea – this may be due to apprehension and anxiety about the acupuncture treatment. An acupuncture point exists to treat nausea if this becomes a recurring problem – P6.
- Dizziness/fainting – patients should initially be treated lying on a bed or couch in case of vasovagal reactions or transient hypotension.
- Drowsiness – up to 9% of patients feel drowsy during or after the first treatment (Filshie & Hester 2006). Warnings must be given about driving home after treatments. However, drowsiness generally decreases gradually with repeated treatments.
- Nerve irritation – caution is required not to pierce or damage nerve tissue during deep needling. Such injuries are rare; however, needling around the fibular head (GB34 point) has resulted in complete paralysis of the nerve and foot drop has been reported in at least one case (Sobel *et al.* 1997, cited in Ernst & White 1999).
- Broken or bent needle – needles must be inspected before use and any bent or suspect needles discarded. Patients may move during the time when the needle is left in place, instruction is needed to prevent needle being pushed in further by the patients' movements. Needle breakage is very rare with the advent of disposable pre-sterilised needles. The weakest area is where the handle joins the shaft; needles should never be completely inserted to the end of the shaft, but rather longer needles selected. Breakage can occur with any forceful insertion or manipulation; the practitioner must ensure any suspicion of breakage is reported as it may require a surgical removal.
- Needle lost or miscounted – when needles are removed, they should be counted and checked against the introducer/packets in the consultation room to ensure that the same number is removed as inserted. Clear documentation to record number used specific areas of the body treated will help ensure needles are not missed and left in the patient.

The practice of acupuncture is not risk free; however, avoidance of predictable adverse events can be minimised by appropriate training and local guidelines to support practice, as discussed later. This is supported by Kaptchuk (2002), who discusses 'the combined data from prospective and retrospective studies that indicate acupuncture is a very safe intervention in the hands of a competent practitioner'.

Children

The focus of this chapter is acupuncture in adults; however, it would not be complete without mentioning the position with children. A factor to consider is that children are generally afraid of needles and acupuncture involves insertion of fine gauge needles. Kemper *et al.* (2000) study showed 'that paediatric patients with chronic pain that was unresponsive to mainstream treatments found acupuncture pleasant and helpful'. It has been suggested that acupressure could be used as a substitute for needles in children to reduce anxiety (Lao 1996).

Pregnancy

Randomised controlled trials have concluded that acupuncture is an effective treatment for women who experience nausea in early pregnancy (Smith *et al.* 2002). This is supported by Cummings (2003), who states 'medical doctors are always cautious and will generally use one point only (P6) as treatment'. The caution derives from concern that spontaneous pregnancy loss may be attributed to acupuncture by the patient if performed before the event whether there is conclusive evidence for this or not.

Acupuncture has been demonstrated as a useful treatment for back and pelvic pain during pregnancy (Thomas & Napolitano 2000, cited in Cummings 2003). Cummings (2003) states that acupuncture should not be classed as a contraindication in pregnancy and describes a case report where six treatments of acupuncture were given for low back pain before pregnancy was confirmed. The patient wished to carry on treatment as it was the most effective treatment for her pain. He also goes on to say that at the time, there were no case reports of pregnancy-related adverse events attributed to acupuncture and no known cases of litigation. The inclusion of pregnant women in the service requires careful consideration of patient suitability if any doubt about potential side effects (Myatt 2005). The most important thing is that the woman is well informed of the state of the evidence and consented appropriately.

Impact on other services

Many patients may seek acupuncture as a treatment when other conventional treatments have failed and may not be trusted due to their inability to provide a 'cure' (Burman 2003). Patients receiving acupuncture that is effective at reducing chronic pain and providing an enhanced sense of well-being may choose the option of fewer medical treatments such as epidural injections, or take regular prescribed medication due to onset of side effects.

Ratcliffe *et al.* (2006) state 'acupuncture treatment for persistent non-specific low back pain confers a modest benefit to health, as measured by quality adjusted life years (QALYs), at relatively minor extra cost to the NHS compared with usual care'. This is supported by Heller (2004), who states 'people who use complementary therapies are often enthusiastic about them and expect access through NHS services'. As a result innovative and imaginative solutions are needed to allow NHS budgets to incorporate such treatments.

The same patient may wish to have regular treatments of acupuncture, which will require an appointment system with regular sessions and flexibility. This needs planning and managing to ensure patients can gain access in a timely manner rather than having to wait for extended periods between treatments.

Integrating acupuncture into mainstream services is difficult when orthodox treatments are evidence based and are provided through statutory health care. However, the roles of 'consumer groups' that use the service are gaining more encouragement with stronger government support (Heller 2004).

Consideration must be given to the long-term impact of such a service on existing services. Can the existing service really support an acupuncture clinic longer term? Are there adequate resources to provide both the existing and acupuncture services? If not what parts of the current service will be lost to provide it and which has the stronger evidence base of clinical effectiveness? If the service is going to be underresourced, the question must be asked: Is it really in the patients and communities best interest to develop a new acupuncture service?

Types of pain

Increasing evidence from systematic reviews are starting to show that acupuncture can be effective for the treatment of headache, fibromyalgia, osteoarthritis of the knee, epicondylitis and low back pain (Filshie & Hester 2006). The service may be developed and triaged to those conditions with the stronger clinical evidence as a way to decrease oversubscription.

Acupuncture is used to treat a variety of chronic pain conditions, as outlined below with the brief evidence available:

- Headache – migraine, tension or cluster. A randomised controlled trial by Coeytaux *et al.* (2005) demonstrated 'that a course of acupuncture treatments improved clinical outcomes among patients with chronic daily headaches beyond what would be expected from speciality medical management treatments'.
- Fibromyalgia – generally fibromyalgia has not been supported through trials founding it of no real benefit over placebo (White *et al.* 2006). This is often conflicted by patient reports that verbalise general benefits such as positive sleep and mood effects impacting on their quality of life.
- Osteoarthritis of the knee – Tukmachi *et al.* (2004) showed 'that manual and electroacupuncture causes a significant improvement in the symptoms of osteoarthritis of the knee, either on its own or as an adjunct therapy'.
- Epicondylitis – a study by Fink *et al.* (2002) demonstrated 'that acupuncture with correct location and stimulation according to TCM seems to alleviate pain and improve function in epicondylitis'.
- Low back pain – Brinkhaus *et al.* (2006) demonstrated evidence 'that patients with chronic back pain who receive acupuncture experience clinically relevant benefits compared with patients who received no acupuncture'.
- Cervical and shoulder pain – a study by Ga et al. (2007) compared acupuncture needling to injecting lidocaine into trigger points situated around the trapezius muscles of the neck. This concluded that patients developed reduced long-term pain and greater range of movements in the elderly participants having acupuncture.

- Facial pain – trigeminal neuralgia, temporomandibular pain – a study by Smith *et al.* (2007) demonstrated that acupuncture had a positive influence on the outcomes of temporomandibular joint myofascial pain compared to 'sham' acupuncture.

Treatment pathways

The treatment pathways for acupuncture are varied without good-quality evidence on which to base the services. The course and frequency of treatment sessions varies according to patient preference, provider beliefs, e.g. western or eastern approach, and resource available. A patient paying for treatment privately may decide to access treatment more or less frequently according to their ability to pay, whereas a patient may continue to have treatment, despite little benefit, if receiving it within the NHS. It is important when considering setting up a service to take into account all of the above factors and make sure that treatment sessions are evaluated to ensure efficacy and the most appropriate treatment pathways for the individual. It is also important to remember that acupuncture is a part of the patients' overall pain management plan and fragmentation of services, i.e. patients having to move between providers for parts of their treatment, e.g. accessing acupuncture privately from one provider and attending for other pain interventions simultaneously with another provider, which can cause confusion, duplication and unnecessary complications.

The core components of an adequate protocol seem to be attention to the number of needles used, the needling technique, specific elicitation of a needling sensation, the number of treatment sessions and the experience of the acupuncturist (White *et al.* 2008).

The majority of pain services within the UK provide a combination of acupuncture courses and 'one-offs' or single top-up sessions. These are briefly described below.

Treatment courses

Patients are generally offered a course of acupuncture with one treatment per week over 4–6 weeks. White *et al.* (2008) describe 'the effects of acupuncture are complex and more than simply needling specific areas with individualistic plans of treatment including lifestyle advice'. This should be built into the initial development process. The study went on to propose 'the definition of dose as the physical procedures using one or more needles, an account of the patients responses (sensory, motor, affective and cognitive), different doses are needed for different conditions'. The study concluded that research is needed into what constitutes an adequate dose of acupuncture. Treatment goals should be pain relief/reduction without adverse side effects and improvement of the patients' well-being, activity and sleep.

The acupuncturist will assess the patient's pain and decide on the appropriate area to treat and number of needles required at the first session. Needles are placed into the skin and left in position for between 10 and 20 minutes depending on the patient's response. Campbell (1998) states 'stimulation of the needles may be used by some acupuncturists. Manual stimulation is applied by rotating, lifting and lowering the needles in the tissues. The decision to use stimulation is an individual matter and acupuncturist's opinions will vary'. Patients may report aggravation of pain after overstimulation and have a reduced therapeutic response. Kong *et al.* (2002) demonstrated 'results have been found using functional MRI (magnetic resonance imaging) that demonstrates how acupuncture stimulation can modulate the activity of the limbic system and other neural activity'. Such information may help refine acupuncture treatment protocols to achieve maximum clinical efficacy; however, the authors of this research conclude that far more work is needed to investigate the correlation between brain activity patterns and acupuncture stimulation.

Whilst the needles are in position, the patient is generally given a selection of relaxation music and covered with a sheet or gown to maintain dignity and retain body heat. Patient positioning is paramount to help relaxation and comfort – either lying on a couch or sitting on recliner chairs.

A number of patients will develop temporary increased pain at the first session and these patients often continue to require courses of treatments to allow their initial increased pain response to develop into an overall pain reduction. Interestingly, these patients will often state the pain reduction does not become noticeable until the third or fourth week of the course. Such changes can be monitored using recognised pain tools and clinical question and answering techniques to assess the patient's pain reduction alongside increased activity levels, quality-of-life indicators and any reduction in the amount of analgesia required.

The clinician discusses the risks and benefits of acupuncture and a patient information leaflet is provided for them to take away. Clear explanation is always given that acupuncture is not a 'cure' for their pain. However, there are a number of patients who develop a very positive response immediately. This needs further study to gain understanding, as pain reduction may be due to a number of factors other than the acupuncture itself – the environment and ambiance of the clinic, confidence with the acupuncturist, the extra help and support they receive regarding lifestyle and medications or even the access to someone who seems to understand their pain.

Top-ups or one-offs

These are single acupuncture treatments generally suitable for patients who experience pain reduction immediately following their first session of a course. The same principles apply in relation to assessment, number of needles, length of time in situ and patient comfort and positioning as discussed above. Generally 'top-ups' are provided around every 8–10 weeks.

The lack of agreement of what is an adequate acupuncture treatment will always be an obstacle to good patient care and further research (White *et al.* 2008). However, a decision will have to be made regarding the type and number of sessions the service will provide locally.

Here lies an extremely difficult situation and it becomes hard to find a solution that meets each individual patient's expectations. White *et al.* (2008) clearly state 'clinical experience strongly suggests that responders and non-responders exist and this has long been recognised in animal studies and may have a genetic basis'. Resources are limited throughout the NHS and acupuncture is not without potential complications; therefore, if patients are unable to describe any difference in their chronic pain, quality-of-life indicators or general increased sense of well-being, then acupuncture will be unsuccessful and not repeated.

This can be very difficult for patients to accept as they may have had unrealistic expectations from either other health professionals or family members regarding the success of acupuncture or the potential longevity of treatment. Setting standards and devising policies to evaluate the effectiveness of individual treatments can provide objective assessment and equitable access to the limited resource.

Staff development: education and maintaining competencies

Recent shifts in the public's perception of the health care professions has led to the expectation that patients and clients are no longer passive recipients of care but equal partners who demand knowledge and agreed standards of education and practice from health care professionals. For health care practitioners, governance and professional regulation is now focused on patient safety and patient choice. The setting and monitoring of standards for education and continuing professional development (CPD) means that health care practitioners are now required to document and provide evidence of their learning. These documents provide the evidence for the knowledge and competence to provide safe, evidence-based care for patients and clients. However, there has been little pressure on complementary medicine practitioners or organisations to reach or provide set standards of education (Mills 2001).

Foundation training

Education of health care practitioners who practise acupuncture will vary depending on the area in which they work and this is reflected in the *Statutory Regulation of the Acupuncture Profession*, the report of the Acupuncture Regulatory Working Group (2003), which found that acupuncture education reflects the diversity of professional contexts in which acupuncture is practised within the UK. There is also variation in the approaches to education and CPD of different professional groups.

Acupuncture programmes of study vary in content, academic level and application. The choice of foundation training for nurses wishing to practise acupuncture for pain management should be carefully considered. Many complementary medicine organisations offer courses of study, and these organisations are recognised as equivalent to professional bodies. They publish codes of ethics and practice that are accepted by health care professionals and the NHS. However, the current situation of self-regulation may not be tenable, and organisations may soon be required to develop more rigorous standards and objectives in the programmes of education they offer (Mills 2001). Some courses offered are medical in emphasis and content and based on the Western philosophies of health care. Others may provide courses of study that are based on the traditional Chinese approach to acupuncture. A balanced approach is essential (Shifrin 1995), and educational programmes should have emphasis on the context in which acupuncture is practised. A suggested core syllabus for any

Table 6.1 Suggested core syllabus for any programme of study for the application of acupuncture by nurses in a chronic pain clinic

- Global history and philosophy of acupuncture
- Understanding health and ill-health
- Knowledge of causes and presentations of chronic pain and common pain syndromes
- Assessment skills
- Knowledge of acupuncture points
- Needle selection and insertion techniques
- Stimulation techniques
- A workable knowledge base of anatomy and physiology
- Indications for treatment
- Contraindications to treatment
- Risks
- Patient medications
- Care planning
- Professional responsibilities
- Ethics
- Evidence base and best practice
- Policy development
- Service development
- Continuing professional development
- Knowledge of resources and sources of information

programme of study for the application of acupuncture by nurses in a chronic pain clinic is outlined in Table 6.1.

Although the underpinning theoretical knowledge is essential, it should be remembered that acupuncture is a practical skill, and any programme of education should include a large component of practical application to enable students to apply theories and techniques learned in the classroom to practise.

Supervisors on these programmes of study should be experienced practitioners who have wide knowledge and experience of the application of acupuncture, and of supervision and mentorship of health care professionals. Students undertaking acupuncture courses are often inexperienced and anxious at first when assessing patients and practising their acupuncture skills; therefore, confident, expert supervision is essential to enable practitioners to develop competence and expertise.

Nursing and other health care professionals have adopted the development of portfolios as a method of documenting and assessing practice in the last decade (Ball *et al.* 2000). There is continuing debate about whether this method of reflecting on and documenting practice provides evidence of learning and professional development; however, it is generally accepted that structured and supervised construction of a portfolio enables students to critically reflect on and develop their practice, and this may be appropriate for students of acupuncture.

To overcome the problem of relevance to the specific health care setting and professional issues in nursing, specialist nurses in some pain management services have designed and delivered courses 'in-house'. These courses of study have been supported and accredited by a higher education institution that is able to provide academic guidance and standards on theoretical components of the course and any assignments, portfolio development and assessments of practice undertaken by students and supervisors during the programme of study. It is possible to develop programmes of study that are holistic in approach and balanced educationally to provide knowledge of philosophies on complementary therapies and their place in modern health care, including traditional Chinese and Western practice and theories in medicine. On completion of foundation training, practitioners are then able to apply knowledge of all theories and traditions that govern the practice of acupuncture to achieve optimum evidence-based care for patients and clients.

The possibility of future regulation of practitioners of complementary therapies has resulted in a reduction of choice for many practitioners over the type of programme of study they wish to undertake, as there is currently uncertainty surrounding how regulation of practitioners and education, and how standards will be set and monitored. Until there is more clarity, established organisations will continue to be the only option for new practitioners to access education as possible alternative providers wait for the outcome of the work of the DH Steering Group from May 2008.

Continuing professional development

This section explores the importance of the educational preparation to prepare practitioners undertaking acupuncture. The role of interprofessional learning in this is also discussed.

The support and mentorship of already qualified practitioners is important, as many students experience anxiety initially as they may feel that they lack knowledge on issues such as point and needle selection and insertion. However, this can be overcome by providing supervision from experienced practitioners. Experienced nurse specialists are often able to offer support and supervision for the practice and development of acupuncture for pain management. Networking between pain management services can be a useful way to gain support and supervision for practice.

Professional development, professional issues and professional relationships are an important element of any programme of study for nursing practice. The *Code of Professional Conduct* (NMC 2004) states that practitioners must act at all times in the best interests of the patient. It is the responsibility of all registered practitioners to ensure that their skills are current and fit for purpose (NMC 2004). Therefore, it is the responsibility of the practitioner to remain competent to practice by updating their knowledge through reading literature and seeking supervision to update practical skills. This is equally important for experienced practitioners who will be providing supervision and support as for students and new practitioners.

Nurses practising acupuncture should give careful consideration to the education and CPD of all health care practitioners who will be working in the area. This will generally be registered nurses, but in some acupuncture clinics, health care assistants may be carrying out duties such as removing and disposing of needles, and the educational needs of this group of workers must also be addressed. This will include issues such as infection control, health and safety legislation, policies and procedures, as well as patient care and well-being. Registered practitioners must accept that they remain accountable for any duties that they delegate to unregistered health care workers.

It is vital that senior clinicians and managers of pain services provide the culture, environment and structure for CPD to be practised and provided (Price 2007). Practitioners of acupuncture should be given the opportunity to continually develop their skills and knowledge in a safe learning environment that positively encourages personal and professional development and which in turn will lead to excellent, evidence-based practice. Development of practice through research and audit is also an important consideration, and CPD should also include education to enable practitioners to implement research and audit projects to support service development.

In line with current policy (DH 2001), the concept and culture of lifelong learning will become increasingly important within the NHS (Tait & Cummings 2004) and are seen as an integral part of CPD (Howatson-Jones 2003). The need to develop lifelong learners is seen as imperative to the delivery of clinically effective care by staff who are able to think, reflect and demonstrate their professional development (Gill 2007). The educational needs of staff are changing, and any new regulatory framework will need to take into account that traditional methods of delivery of programmes of learning may not be appropriate in the twenty-first century. An example of modernising education and professional development may be designing of e-learning packages (Gill 2007), which are flexible and take into account different learning styles and circumstances of students.

Interprofessional learning and working

The original working group (Acupuncture Regulatory Working Group 2003) states that any regulation must not limit the use of acupuncture to the extent that the current drive towards interprofessional learning and practice (DH 2001) is limited. The concept of interprofessional learning seems to be particularly relevant to the practice of complementary medicine as, particularly within the NHS, complementary therapies are rarely practised in isolation, and professional groups will need to develop methods of learning and working together to enable delivery of clinically and economically effective, evidence-based practice which has the patient or client at the centre of their care. The philosophies of shared care and collaboration between professions inherent in the concept of interprofessional learning and working (DH 2001) and their relevance to clinical practice continue to be poorly understood (Kenny 2002), but the opportunities for the concept to improve understanding and relationships between the professions, and so increasing service user partnership, participation and effectiveness of care are in keeping with the philosophies underpinning the learning, practice and development of complementary therapies.

Clinical governance

The final section of this chapter considers the importance of clinical governance and how policies and procedures need to be developed to provide a robust framework to support acupuncture services. According to the NHS Clinical Governance Support Team, 'clinical governance is the framework that helps organizations provide safe and high quality care' and 'brings together all the activity that contributes to the clinical service provided to patients.'

They also suggest that the key characteristics of ideal health care are that it should be 'safe, effective, patient-centered, timely, efficient and equitable' (NHS Clinical Governance Support Team, http://www.hqip.org.uk/clinical-audit-handbook/, accessed February 2009). These characteristics aim to avoid injuries, are based on scientific knowledge, should consider individual preferences and should provide the same quality of care to all, regardless of age, gender or ability to pay.

These characteristics obviously apply to any patient care situation, but this will focus on the implementation of clinical governance standards when setting up an acupuncture clinic for chronic pain management.

Prior to setting up the clinic in a new setting it is important to ensure that there is a robust system of clinical governance in place. Clinical governance will incorporate patient information, consent, policies and procedures, as well as a complaints system that is easily accessible. These systems ensure that patients are safe when undergoing their treatment and need to be proactive. It is not an acceptable practice to wait for something to go wrong before ensuring that there is a system in place to be able to deal with it, but can also help in the prevention of an untoward incident occurring in the first instance.

Policies and procedures

There are several policies that should be considered prior to setting up the service. Some suggestions could be:

- How long the treatment will continue if the patient has had any benefit from it. It is important to ascertain from the outset whether the service will provide acupuncture treatment indefinitely, or whether the acupuncture will be given for a set number of treatments, with a plan for future care.
- The referral process to the service, including who can refer, and which patients could be referred. In this policy it is important to stipulate that the acupuncture is only performed for patients who have chronic pain.
- Procedures should cover aspects such as:
  - technique
  - training
  - practice development and practice updates.

All policies and procedures will need to be ratified by the clinical governance team responsible for the trust to ensure that all parties are protected. The building blocks of a sound governance framework will incorporate attention to audit procedures, documentation, patient information, consent, safety/risks, insurance, patient complaints and communications.

Audit

Audit has an essential part to play in setting up an acupuncture clinic. Audit is one way of being able to find out what patients feel about their care, as well as being able to specifically identify any common themes or problems that may occur. Many tools are available to audit the service including assessment and evaluation questionnaires and computer software based on pain levels and quality-of-life indicators.

Documentation

Another aspect of patient safety is documentation. Again there must be clear guidance about the format of the documentation and what is the most appropriate way of documenting the patient care. It is important that everyone agrees on the format, whether there will be a generic form, or if the staff feel that it is more appropriate to write each patient episode individually.

Patient information

Patient information is of vital importance. This must be clearly written, easy to understand and of good quality. The information that the patient receives must highlight the way that the treatment is thought to work, as well as the risks and benefits of acupuncture. This will help in the process of gaining informed consent. Consideration must be made regarding the format and language of the information provided based on the diversity of the local community. Patient reader panels are key in this process.

Consent

It is obviously important to gain patient consent prior to the treatment starting. Again, clear guidelines must be agreed on the format that the consent will take. There needs to be liaison with the appropriate clinical governance and patient safety teams to ensure best practice in gaining consent. Is it acceptable to assume that if the patient has attended for their appointment, has undressed and is lying in a position then that would lead the health care professional to think that the patient wanted the acupuncture treatment? Or, is it more appropriate to set up a system of gaining written consent when the patient attends for the treatment? This issue must be clarified with clinical governance.

Insurance

If all policies and procedures are ratified by clinical governance and are adhered to during practice, the acupuncturist is protected by vicarious liability through their employing body.

Safety and risk assessments

The safety and risk assessments must include ensuring that the actual environment is safe and appropriate to carry out treatment. It must also include assessments to ensure that the acupuncturist can ascertain that they can work in a safe environment. The acupuncturist can potentially spend a lot of time on their own, during the assessment and treatment of the patient, and if the acupuncturist feels in any way threatened by the patient, they need to know that they can raise help, if needed. The environment also needs to be patient-friendly. By nature of chronic pain, the patients who attend for acupuncture may have substantially reduced mobility, so the department needs to establish ways in which patients can access the department and the treatment areas. It is important to be able to provide a safe and comfortable environment for all people attending the department.

Complaints system

The Government has produced a toolkit ensuring good practice in managing complaints at a local level (Department of Health, 2009). Again, although this is for all aspects of the NHS, it can be applied to an acupuncture service. Complaints about the service should not be seen as a threat, but should be seen as a way of gaining feedback and making improvements when able. The complaints system should be easily accessible to all.

Liaison and communications

An accessible complaints system should be part of a wider communications system between the service provider and the service user. It is important that patients have the opportunity to comment on aspects of the service that they feel are helpful as well as areas for improvement. This can be achieved by providing a focus group, which is a group of five to eight, facilitated by a member of staff, preferably someone who does not provide the acupuncture service. Focus groups can take the format of a conversation, and one benefit of this is that patients can discuss various aspects which they feel important, as they are led by comments which other patients make. The facilitator must be skilled in making sure that one person does not take over the whole session, therefore not allowing others to have their say. It is also important to ensure that patients do not use the group as a way of venting their anger, or grievance to a captured audience, so it is important that the facilitator lays down ground rules before the conversation starts. Ideas or points raised during the discussion are then recorded and fed back to the service providers. They can then be acted on, where appropriate. To ensure that the patient is kept at the centre of their care, there must be a robust system of communication between the service provider, the patient's general practitioner, the referrer (if different from the general practitioner) and any other relevant health care worker.

Although acupuncture is relatively safe and has few contraindications, it must be viewed as a treatment modality alongside medications or invasive procedures. Because of this, all health care providers should be made aware that their patient is receiving this form of treatment so that it can be viewed as part of a package of treatment for chronic pain.

Conclusions

The development of any new service requires careful consideration of the political, clinical and governance issues; therefore, advanced skills are required to understand and manage the complexity of issues during negotiation and implementation of such services. The development of an acupuncture service in the current climate requires all these skills and more. The nurse must be aware of the current funding pathways and ensure that the service is sustainable and appropriately placed linking into existing services to serve the best interests of the clients. The educational aspects of staff training and development are crucial for the development and maintenance of the service. This is of particular importance currently as mandatory registration for acupuncture is, as discussed earlier, a hot political debate. Careful consideration must also be taken to identify the potential risks of the service and systems put in place to minimise those risks and record and manage any untoward incidents.

Editors' note

This chapter takes a slightly different stance by providing an overview of developing an acupuncture service for people with pain. The lead author initially developed the service but later worked with others as they developed their own services. It emphasises the importance of not only developing a service, but sharing best practice and supporting others to develop new services. The importance of providing coaching, mentoring and consultancy for other colleagues to facilitate their service development reflects yet another level for those involved in advanced practitioner.

References

Acupuncture Regulatory Working Group, 2003. *The Statutory Regulation of the Acupuncture Profession*. London: Prince of Wales Foundation for Integrated Health.

Ball, E., Daly, W.M., Carnwell, R., 2000. The use of portfolios in the assessment of learning and competence. *Nursing Standard*, 14(43), 35–37.

Brinkhaus, B., Witt, C.W., Jenna, S., Linde, K., Streng, A., Wagenpfeil, S., Irnich, D., Heinz-Ulrich, W., Melchart, D., Willich, S., 2006. Acupuncture in patients with chronic low back pain – a randomised controlled trial. *Archives of Internal Medicine*, 166, 450–457.

Burman, M.C., 2003. Complementary and alternative medicine: core competencies for family nurse practitioners. *Journal of Nursing Education*, 42(1), 28–34.

Campbell, A., 1998. Methods of acupuncture. In Filshie, J., White, A. (eds), *Medical Acupuncture – A Western Scientific Approach*. p 19–32. Edinburgh: Churchill Livingstone.

Coeytaux, R., Kaufman, J.S., Kaptchuk, T.J., Chen, W., Miller, W.C., Callahan, L.F., Mann, D., 2005. A randomised controlled trial of acupuncture for chronic daily headache. *Headache*, 45, 1113–1123.

Cummings, M., 2003. Acupuncture for low back pain in pregnancy. *Acupuncture in Medicine*, 21(1–2), 42–46.

Department of Health, 2001. *Working Together – Learning Together: A Framework for Lifelong Learning for the NHS*. London: HMSO.

Department of Health Steering Group, 2008. *Report to Ministers from The Department of Health Steering Group on the Statutory Regulation of Practitioners of Acupuncture, Herbal Medicine, Traditional Chinese Medicine and Other Traditional Medicine Systems Practiced in the UK*. London: DH.

Drug and Therapeutics Bulletin, 2007. Acupuncture for osteoarthritis of the knee. *Drug and Therapeutics Bulletin*, 45, 76–79.

Filshie, J., Hester, J., 2006. Guidelines for providing acupuncture treatment for cancer patients – a peer reviewed sample policy document. *Acupuncture in Medicine*, 24(4), 172–182.

Fink, M., Wolkenstein, E., Karst, M., Gehrke, A., 2002. Acupuncture in chronic epicondylitis: a randomised controlled trial. *Rheumatology*, 41(2), 205–209.

Fujiwara, H., Taniguchi, K., Takeuchi, J., Ikezono, E., 1980. The influence of low frequency acupuncture on a demand pacemaker. Cited in Norris, C. (ed.) 2004. *Acupuncture – Treatment of Musculoskeletal Conditions*. Oxford: Butterworth Heinemann.

Ga, H., Choi, J.H., Park, C.H., Yoon, H.J., 2007. Acupuncture needling versus lidocaine injection of trigger points in myofascial pain syndrome in elderly patients – a randomised controlled trial. *Acupuncture in Medicine*, 25(4), 130–136.

Gill, A., 2007. E-learning and professional development – never too old to learn. *British Journal of Nursing*, 16(17), 1084–1088.

Department of Health, 2009. Handling complaints in the NHS – good practice toolkit for local resolution. Available at http://www.dh.gov.uk/en/Publicationsandstatistics/Publications/PublicationsPolicyAndGuidance/Browsable/DH_5133738 [accessed 25 February 2009].

Heller, T., 2004. Integrating complementary and alternative medicine. *Nursing Management*, 11(7), 32–37.

Hopwood, V., Lovesey, M., Mokone, S., 1997. *Acupuncture* and related techniques in physical therapy, p. 126. Oxford: Churchill Livingstone.

Howatson-Jones, I., 2003. Difficulties in clinical supervision and lifelong learning. *Nursing Standard*, 17(37), 37–41.

Kaptchuk, T.J., 2002. Acupuncture: theory, efficacy and practice. *Annals of Internal Medicine*, 136(5), 374–383.

Kemper, K.J., Sarah, R., Silver-Highfield, E., Xiarhos, E., Barnes, L., Berde, C., 2000. Complementary and alternative medicine: on pins and needles? Pediatric patients experience with acupuncture. *Pediatrics*, 105(4, Pt 2), 941–947.

Kenny, G., 2002. Interprofessional working: opportunities and challenges. *Nursing Standard*, 17(6), 33–35.

Kong, J., Ma, L., Gollub, R.L., Wei, J., Yang, X., Li, D., Weng, X., Jia, F., Wang, C., Li, F., Li, R., Zhuang, D., 2002. A study of functional magnetic resonance imaging of the brain during manual and electroacupuncture stimulation of acupuncture point (LI-4 Hegu) in normal subjects reveals differential brain activation between methods. *The Journal of Alternative and Complementary Medicine*, 8(4), 411–419.

Lao, L., 1996. Acupuncture techniques and devices. *Journal of Alternative Complementary Medicine*, 2, 23–25.

Mills, S.Y., 2001. Regulation in complementary and alternative medicine. *British Medical Journal*, 322, 158–160.

Myatt, A., 2005. Exploring the therapeutic effects of acupuncture. *Nursing and Residential Care*, 7(11), 513–515.

Norris, C., 2001. *Acupuncture* – Treatment of Musculoskeletal Conditions. Oxford: Butterworth Heinemann.

Nursing and Midwifery Council, 2004. *Code of Professional Conduct: Standards for Conduct, Performance and Ethics*. London: NMC.

Price, B., 2007. Professional development opportunities in changing times. *Nursing Standard*, 12(25), 29–33.

Ratcliffe, J., Thomas, K.J., MacPherson, H., Brazier, J., 2006. A randomised controlled trial of acupuncture care for persistent low back pain: cost effectiveness analysis. *BMJ*, 333, 626.

Shifrin, K., 1995. Squaring the circle: the core syllabus of the British Acupuncture Accreditation Board. *Complementary Therapies in Medicine*, 3, 13–15.

Smith, C., Crowther, C., Beilby, J., 2002. Acupuncture to treat nausea and vomiting in early pregnancy:a randomised controlled trial. *Birth*, 29, 1–9.

Smith, P., Mosscrop, D., Davies, S., Sloan, P., Al-Ani, Z., 2007. The efficacy of acupuncture in the treatment of temporomandibular joint myofascial pain: a randomised controlled trial. *Journal of Dentistry*, 35(3), 259–267.

Sobel, E., Huang, E., Weiting, C., 1997. Drop foot as a complication of acupuncture injury and intragluteal injection. Cited in Ernst, E., White, A. (eds), 1999. *Acupuncture – A Scientific Approach*. Oxford: Butterworth-Heinemann.

Tait, J., Cummings, M., 2004. Education, training and continuing professional development in medical acupuncture – a contemporary overview. *Acupuncture in Medicine*, 22(2), 75–82.

Thomas, C.T., Napolitano, P.G., 2000. Use of acupuncture for managing chronic pelvic pain in pregnancy. A case report. Cited in Cummings, M. (ed.), 2003. Acupuncture for low back pain in pregnancy. *Acupuncture in Medicine*, 21(1–2), 42–46.

Thomas, K.J., MacPherson, H., Thorpe, L., Brazier, J., Fitter, M., Campbell, M.J., Roman, M., Walters, S.J., Nicholl, J., 2006. Randomised controlled trial of a short course of traditional acupuncture compared with usual care for persistent non-specific low back pain. *BMJ online*, 333, 623.

Thomas, K.S., Nicoll, J.P., Coleman, P.C., 2001. Use and expenditure on complementary medicine in England: a population based survey. *Complementary Therapies in Medicine*, 9, 2–11.

Tsuei, J.J., Lee, Y.-F., Sharma, S.D., 1977. The influence of acupuncture stimulation during pregnancy. The induction and inhibition of labour. *Obstetrics and Gynecology*, 50, 479–488.

Tukmachi, E., Jubb, R., Dempsey, E., Jones, P., 2004. The effect of acupuncture on the symptoms of knee osteoarthritis – an open randomised controlled study. *Acupuncture in Medicine*, 22(1), 14–22.

White, A., Cummings, M., Barlas, P., Cardini, F., Filshie, J., Foster, N.E., Lundeberg, T., Sterner-Victorin, E., Witt, C., 2008. Defining an adequate dose of acupuncture using a neurophysiological approach – a narrative review of the literature. *Acupuncture in Medicine*, 26(2), 111–120.

White, A., Tough, E., Cummings, M., 2006. A review of acupuncture clinical trials indexed during 2005. *Acupuncture in Medicine*, 24(1), 39–49.

Chapter 7
The advanced nurse practitioner: developing alliances

Ruth Day and Dee Burrows

Introduction

The provision of services in the health sector in the UK is changing rapidly. The advanced nurse practitioner (ANP) is in a position to influence, and be influenced by, this evolving landscape. This chapter explores how some of these services have developed and considers the challenges and opportunities presented. This is done by using models from the business sector, particularly those that consider the role of the entrepreneur within the development of alliances. The vignettes presented will show how the competencies of ANPs place them in an enviable position to develop alliances. Throughout the chapter the challenges facing nurses who are looking to develop services in this way will be faced. Finally, a number of key resources are identified.

Alliances and strategic alliances

An alliance can be described as an agreement between two or more people (or groups) to enable them to work towards something they have in common. A strategic alliance is seen within the business world where two or more companies make a formal agreement to harness 'each other's core competencies in order that each can maximize the opportunity to implement their strategic intent' (Adams 2001).

Strategic alliances are rapidly becoming a method of joint venturing used widely in the business world, growing rapidly since the 1970s. In essence they are partnerships in which businesses combine their efforts in 'a business-to-business collaboration' (Kautz 2008). Strategic alliances rely upon establishing business networks and are a model used by many large companies, such as the airline industry. In health care – particularly in the USA – alliances have been formed between clinicians, academics and the pharmaceutical industry (Kennedy & Bormann 2006). Within the NHS we have seen large-scale alliances within PFI (private finance initiative) projects. However, the underlying approaches are not constrained to large business. Entrepreneurial nurses can adapt and use many of the methods in developing new and innovative services both within and out with the NHS.

Changing workplaces

The last 10 years has been a time of great change in the politics and service provision of the NHS. There are openings for nurses to manage services in primary care, to work autonomously in walk-in centres and to set up their own businesses, some becoming partners in business with GPs (Crombie 2006). It is probably within primary care that change has been the most obvious. To some extent this is not surprising, as GPs are private contractors to the NHS, but big, multinational companies are now bidding for GP service contracts from PCTs. This is producing a very mixed response from health care professionals and patients (Arie 2006). However, with changes in purchasing, the opportunities for developing new ways of delivering pain services have never been greater. One example within the NHS is in the growing development of ANPs or nurse consultants taking the lead in moving chronic pain services into primary care from their traditional place in secondary care, as seen in other chapters in this book. There is also an expansion of pain services within the independent sector (Burrows 2006). Private health care facilities (such as BMI hospitals) have often provided an interventional chronic pain service but few, if any, provide a full range of pain services. The recent expansion of independent pain services has begun to address this gap.

Skill acquisition

What skills are needed to identify gaps in service and advance practice in this way? Wallace (2004) suggests that there are four areas in which skills should be developed (see Table 7.1).

The UK nursing literature has much on leadership – mostly within clinical situations – but little on entrepreneurship or the development of alliances. This lack of literature was noted by Traynor *et al.* (2006) who state 'the international empirically based literature on this topic is very small suggesting that many aspects have not been objectively examined. The narrative and descriptive accounts by entrepreneurial nurses are more common but not extensive' (p. 72). However, many of the skills described

Table 7.1 Skills development based on Wallace (2004)

1	Know yourself	Maximise your ability and capacity to do work and perform tasks – *analyse your own organisation*
2	Know your plan	Develop a bridge to close the gap between the present and a future entrepreneurial venture – *planning is essential*
3	Know your universe	Maintain harmony between your strategy and the constraints of the area in which you plan to work – *understand the wider environment in which you and your potential partner work*
4	Know your resources and make them your own	Investigate others' successes and failures – *this will increase your odds of being successful*

in nursing literature as 'leadership roles' have a good fit with the categories outlined by Wallace (2004). Perhaps there is something about language here. Do nurses who develop new services see themselves as leaders or as entrepreneurs? We suggest that there is a subtle difference – a leader may take a team into an area which is new for his or her team, but follow a path which has been trodden previously. Conversely, an entrepreneur sees or develops an area which has not been worked in that particular way before. Both will need similar skills – they may both need to develop alliances with others, for example, but the entrepreneur will not have as much guidance available. ANPs certainly need the skills of a leader, but we believe that some will also have the making of an entrepreneur. Hughes *et al.* (2006) identify some of the skills required for entrepreneurship in policy development. These include developing activities that lay the groundwork to allow new concepts and proposals to emerge. They suggest that a key activity is influencing people and events within different organisations and at various levels within these organisations to both use and create opportunities. There is a similarity here with the concept of strategic alliances outlined in our opening paragraph.

The report by Traynor *et al.* (2006) suggests that the term entrepreneur is usually associated with the business world and wealth creation. They find an overlap with nurses working as entrepreneurs, as intrapreneurs (an employee who behaves in an entrepreneurial way within their organisation) and social entrepreneurs (those who apply enterprise and imagination to social, rather than wealth, creation). This movement into social enterprise is growing in the NHS, and the King's Fund has suggested that staff who want to compete in these areas may have to develop non-profit-making social enterprises (Arie 2006). Further information about social enterprises can be found via the Social Enterprise Coalition website (http://www.socialenterprise.org.uk/, accessed 25 February 2009). Of note, the coalition defines social enterprise as organisations whose 'aim is to generate profit to further their social and environmental goals' rather than shareholder value. It is possible that in health care, nurse entrepreneurs might incorporate social enterprise activities into profit-making organisations. In other words, the two do not need to be mutually exclusive.

This chapter will use three real-life vignettes to explore how ANPs can enable new ideas to emerge, create opportunities and develop alliances, using intra- and entrepreneurial skills. Their impact will be explored from a variety of perspectives.

Developing entrepreneurial services in pain management

There are a number of nurse-based organisations that can assist nurses thinking about becoming more strategic and entrepreneurial in their outlook. Largest among these is the Royal College of Nursing, which has a Nurse Entrepreneurs Group which is a subgroup of the RCN Nurse Managers Forum. The group meets to offer support, networking and occasional workshops to discuss the practicalities of working independently. There is also a publication 'Nurse entrepreneurs: turning initiative into independence' (RCN, 2007). Although not focused on pain specifically, there is some general practical advice for those thinking of setting up in business or wanting to read more broadly. The group has also developed an online forum to improve and assist with communication and networking amongst members.

More recently *Entreprenurses* has been established. They describe themselves as 'a Community Interest Company which is a type of social enterprise. What that means is we want to change the world and we want to do it in a businesslike and entrepreneurial way.' Further information about this group can be found on their website (http://www.entreprenurses.net/about/index.php, accessed 25 February 2009).

Outside of the nursing world, organisations such as Business Link, local Chambers of Commerce and the Federation of Small Businesses can provide useful support and advice. In addition, associations such as LinkedIn, the Athena Network and Everywoman offer networking opportunities. In the pain world, membership of local, national and international societies and forums are a must for those wanting to consider the formation of alliances to advance practice.

As discussed above, recent changes in the commissioning and delivery of health services make it more feasible for small ventures to provide local services responsive to local need. Alongside this, there are a growing number of empowered patients who research conditions and treatment prior to visiting health care providers. We suggest that this may also have an influence on service provision. Although pain management does not seem to have been a high priority at government level, it is something which is regarded as very high priority at a personal level. Alliances at the local level with empowered patients may well have an impact on service provision by highlighting the need.

Identifying needs

Identifying need is a key component in developing services wherever one finds oneself. Only once the need is perceived is it possible to consider how it might be met and if the new idea will fill the gap. It is this knowledge of 'your universe' that Wallace (2004) suggests is required to maintain harmony between strategy and constraints. For instance, in the delivery of pain management services a chance conversation might lead you to notice that local care homes have a need for a specific service – say some education for staff about managing residents' pain. Using Wallace's (2004) model you could take a truthful look at yourself and your strengths. Do you have the skills to deliver such education; do you have not only the skills but also the capacity? How would you set about planning it – in practical terms how do you get from A to B? If you continue thinking about it, you need to consider how much you know about the workings of, and the area of, care homes. Is it an area in which you could work in alliance with another organisation? What constraints might there be – or what constraints are already there? What would this symbiotic relationship bring? Who else has been working in the field? What have their successes been and what has ensured them? Have there been any failures and what led to them? What are your chances of success? Some of these questions may be easy to answer and others will take research that may involve others. There will be different answers for different people and situations, but all will give the ANP an opportunity to reflect on the area more closely. It may also be that a development in this kind of health care arena may be considered to be a social enterprise, as defined above. In the vignettes that follow we will show how the various parts of Wallace's model can be seen in use.

Identifying need by audit

Steve (see Vignette 7.1) identified a need when he was looking at current provision. He knew what he and his organisation could deliver. Whilst developing a plan to close the gap between what patients seemed to be saying and what the NHS pain service could offer, he started to think about possible openings and opportunities.

Vignette 7.1

Steve, a consultant nurse in pain management, was tasked with reviewing the chronic pain service. His audit established that patients valued the service but wished they could have accessed it sooner and nearer to home. A subsequent qualitative study formed the basis for a pilot community service. Steve found that the systems and processes, patients and clinicians alike must engage with in order to access and provide chronic pain management, are actually a part of the problem as they almost guarantee physical, social, psychological and spiritual disability. In his attempt to lead a service redesign, he discovered it was almost impossible due to the constraints and priorities that seemed to conspire to create inertia. Yet he had a deep conviction that this was the right thing to do and his determination resulted in the formation of his own independent pain management company. He is now achieving the change in the design of pain management services which patients identified; not in the way he had anticipated, but in a way which has made it possible for the outcomes to be realised.

It was between the step of knowing his plan and knowing his universe that it became clear to Steve that it was impossible to maintain harmony between the strategy (to deliver chronic pain management services in a way which patients identified as helpful) and the constraints of the area in which he was working (trust priorities, workflow patterns, etc.). This disharmony led him back to the drawing board and to consider alternative ways of delivering the service and the patient's need that had been identified. The need did not change, but the perspective did. It became obvious that either one could leave things as they were and not change them, or think about them in a more entrepreneurial manner. Steve felt that in order to provide the service, he believed patients were asking for, he had to look outside the hospital and make alliances with other organisations. His plan changed and the universe he moved into was very unlike the one he knew. PCTs may be part of the NHS, but they function very differently from a specialist area in a hospital. Steve began looking at other models of service provision, seeing what was working, balancing up success and failure before coming to an answer. That answer has led to alliances with other health care providers and, for Steve, a new model of providing for patient's need.

Identifying need from clinical experience

Vignette 7.2

Claire, a pain nurse specialist, manages the inpatient and outpatient pain services in a large district general hospital. Prior to her appointment the two services worked independently. Conjoining them has led to improvements for patients and relatives as well as for staff in the hospital and primary care settings as this case study demonstrates. Jeff is a 72-year-old man known to the outpatient/chronic pain service with low back pain and sciatica secondary to degenerative spinal changes and a disc prolapse. A referral had been made to the orthopaedic team who performed a caudal epidural, which improved his leg pain. Six weeks later he presented to his GP with symptoms that prompted the GP to bleep Claire for advice. Jeff was sent to A&E and subsequently admitted for an urgent scan. Over the next 24 hours his condition deteriorated and his wife rang Claire's voicemail to say she was worried. The ward staff also bleeped the inpatient/acute pain team. As Claire was concerned about Jeff's condition, she reviewed him urgently. The critical care outreach team was called and Jeff was admitted to ITU with sepsis probably due to discitis, although a link with the caudal epidural was not established. Jeff stayed in ITU for 6 weeks. After his discharge from hospital, he and his wife used the voicemail and telephone call back service to access support from the pain team, and he has been seen in outpatients for continuing pain management such as TENS. He is still seeking a cure from surgery and Claire has arranged for an appointment with the orthopaedic team to explain why this is not appropriate.

Claire's experience (Vignette 7.2) is one with which many nurse specialists will have an affinity. The clinical arena depends on good communication with other specialities for the best patient outcomes. The outcomes achieved by Claire were not due to serendipity, but to the foresight of the pain management team in putting in place pathways to facilitate good practice in situations like that experienced by Jeff. In Wallace's (2004) terms the team knew themselves and had put in place systems that enabled them to maximise their capacity. For instance, the voicemail, which relatives could use, enabled the team to make contact when there was the capacity and time to do so. They had analysed their organisation – not the hospital, but their pain service. This shows how the use of a model suggested for entire organisations (large and small) can be used for teams or services within an organisation. The same principles apply. The team's plan to develop a bridge to close the gap between where they were and where they wanted to be had meant that a bleep system for GPs was instigated. Their aim was to provide a seamless service for patients in pain and the strategy they developed included identifying gaps in the system and considering how these might be addressed. Their ability to do so is demonstrated in the successful use of the strategies in Jeff's management.

Identifying a need with a partner

Vignette 7.3 demonstrates a very different way of the development of an entrepreneurial service in pain. Here we see an occasion when a nurse, working in her own company, developed a strategic alliance with industry to research a pain assessment tool for use in primary care.

Vignette 7.3

An independent pain management company, led by Mary, a nurse, was approached to become involved in a project researching the use of a neuropathic pain assessment tool for GPs. They were asked because of proven credibility in pain management and in research. To deliver this multicentre study, links were made with other organisations, such as one providing statistical support and another with skills in protocol development and clinical research management. A team was put in place and the methodology for the project was worked up via email, telephone and face-to-face discussions, through an alliance of the commercial sponsor, experts from other invited organisations and providers led by the nurse. The protocol is being developed within the ethical boundaries set both by professional and personal perspectives and will start data collection in 2008.

In order to achieve this, Mary had to analyse her own organisation, bearing in mind the skills they had which would meet the requirements of the industry partner who had approached her. In considering a joint venture, she had to know the strengths her team could bring (expertise in pain and validation of patient questionnaires, for example) and how her organisation would be able to work with industry to develop the bridge between what was there at present and where they hoped to be. Maintaining harmony between the strategy and the constraints provided some challenges. These necessitated frank discussion and were resolved with some compromise on both sides. Part of the need for the discussions was to enable partners in the alliance to understand the environment in which the other worked and the ethics of each environment. Had there been irreconcilable differences then the project would have foundered.

These three vignettes show how ANPs have developed services within and out with the NHS, and using Wallace's model, various stages can be identified. However, this chapter is about developing alliances, not how to set up services, and the following section will explore further the ways that these people faced the challenges of forming alliances.

The challenge of forming alliances to enable implementation

A considerable number of ANPs develop skills transferable to the arena of entrepreneurism in the way that they manage service redesign and provision within their work areas. However, the question has to be asked whether the associations made, in implementing change or redesigning patient pathways, are actually alliances?

Claire and her team (Vignette 7.2) worked together with other teams in the hospital, but did they do so through the use of alliances? An alliance is the action of combining something, or of forming a union. In one way it would be possible to argue that all health care professionals are in an alliance with each other – our varying disciplines and knowledge combine to form a union of people committed to addressing the needs of our patients. However, this would be broadening, almost to the point of meaninglessness, the usual business understanding of the term. It is more truthful to say that the pain management team worked within a framework of referrals, asking another expert or specialist for advice. At different times during the pathway, Claire was both the referrer and the expert to whom referral was made.

Emerging, embryonic and established

This is not to say that the skills Claire and her team used would not be used in an entrepreneurial project. It is, perhaps, the environment in which they are working that places it within a referral model. Wallace (2004) suggests that there are three categories of entrepreneurs – emerging, embryonic and established. The skills used by Claire (and other ANPs) demonstrate their position as emerging entrepreneurs. They may not become established entrepreneurs, but the skills they use enable the development of services which work towards the establishment of pathways designed to meet an identified need. The people leading these developments could be called intrapreneurs – they are demonstrating entrepreneurial work but from within an organisation.

One of the advantages (or possibly a disadvantage) of being a nurse is that of working in a large profession. The nurses in pain management, who first performed tasks and skills that were the domain of a different health care professional, were intra/entrepreneurs in the broadest sense of the word; but those of us that follow will be unable to claim that. So in this book, you will find examples of current intrapreneurship (for instance, in performing femoral nerve blocks) and areas in which we may follow (for instance, in ordering MRI scans). But within a business model, an entrepreneur is someone who undertakes an enterprise, may own and manage a business and takes the risk of profit or loss.

In this way, although Steve (Vignette 7.1) began the journey as a nurse leader, trying to take a team into a new area, he seems to have finished as an entrepreneur – seeing and developing an area in a new and particular way. This is only one example of a growing number of entrepreneurial activities that are happening in pain management. Some, like Steve's, have been led by nurses; others by different health care professionals. Many of them are multidisciplinary and are building alliances in a variety of areas, often brought into being as a result of constraints within present health care provision. Steve has had to develop alliances with the PCT in order to develop a service for local people in pain.

Vignette 7.3 provides more insight into what a strategic alliance might look like. This vignette demonstrates that one may have to make alliances with more than one party. For example, in order to provide the required input of statistical analysis, Mary had to bring in another partner to deliver on that aspect of the project. As with Claire, where she was at times the referrer and the expert, here Mary is both the smaller company in the project and the controlling one for some aspects of the plan. The approach to Mary by another company indicates that she is moving from the embryonic state to that of an established entrepreneur. She is managing the business and taking the risk of profit (or loss). In acknowledgement of Kautz's (2008) view of strategic alliances as being built on networking and collaborative partnerships, the project described in Vignette 7.3 would not have proceeded in the way it is without the time and skill that Mary and her colleagues have invested in networking in both business and practice arenas. All the partners involved had to be able to recognise the benefits and the strategic 'fit' of the project. Frequently identified benefits in these alliances include ones that are skills related, that lead to cost saving, add value and are market related (Adams 2001). These can be identified in the above vignette and some will relate to one party more than another.

All three of the enterprises included in this chapter demonstrate the application of skills that many ANPs possess, moving beyond the restraints of referral into the freedom of entrepreneurialism. In Vignette 7.2 we perhaps see an emerging entrepreneur, whereas in Vignette 7.1, Steve demonstrates the embryonic stage through developing alliances with and within the PCT to enable him the type of service delivery he identified as more closely fitting with patients expressed needs. In Vignette 7.3 there is some evidence of established entrepreneurship.

Other areas that pain professionals might want to explore include the development of strategic alliances with patients and carers. Earlier we mentioned the possibility of an alliance with empowered patients to influence the provision of service. It may also be feasible to develop alliances with voluntary or charitable groups involved with issues surrounding pain, to work with other health professionals on a shared agenda, to work with commissioning GPs, with occupational health departments in business and so on – the list is only constrained by imagination.

However, in all this excitement, it is important that in making alliances one maintains one's own identity. This is helped by a real understanding of oneself; the first step in Wallace's (2004) outline. The final vignette hinted at the possibility of a conflict of interest, with differences that had to be discussed and compromised upon. What these levels of compromise may be will vary, but in starting to develop alliances we need to ensure that we know how we will maintain our own standards.

The challenge of maintaining standards

Working out how to maintain standards is paramount to successful alliances. At the core of nursing standards is the Nursing and Midwifery Council's (NMC's) code of professional conduct: standards for conduct, performance and ethics. For the ANP, the success of alliances will depend upon maintaining registration and competence in practice, whether clinical, managerial, education or research. An up-to-date professional portfolio evidencing continuing education, professional and business competence and integrity is a must.

It is useful to consider how standards are maintained from a professional and business perspective. These frequently overlap, but for ease we have considered them independently. The areas commented on below are not exhaustive and further help in considering this section more widely can be found in a number of the resources already noted.

Professional

Confidentiality

Some of the tensions that may arise in developing strategic alliances are that the ANP may become party to commercially sensitive information. Successful networking thus relies on an absolute understanding of confidentiality whether project or business related. For example, the RCN's 'Nurse entrepreneurs' publication, previously referred to, highlights the trap of using information databases for reasons other than originally intended – unless the information is already in the public domain.

Trust

It must also be recognised that partnerships, or alliances, do not always work out successfully. Some studies (generally not in health care) have shown that up to 60% fail, or all the parties involved do not feel that the venture was mutually beneficial (Spekman *et al.* 1996). Reasons are manifold, but commonly include a lack of understanding of the differences between the organisations, or that the organisations have very different strategic goals. If there is insufficient trust, or a breakdown in the relationship between key managers in the different organisations, it can render an alliance unworkable. The human factor in alliances may be more influential on the outcome than the business drivers (Adams 2001). This can become an issue when two or more parties are involved (Duysters *et al.* 1999). Ensuring excellent communications and networks are in place is essential. Spending time on this (as in Vignette 7.3) is time well spent so that trust and personal integrity is established.

Business

Insurance

A variety of insurances are required by us all in both our personal and professional lives. What these include are specific to the individual context, but in terms of nursing practice we all need professional indemnity insurance. This is something that most of us, firmly embedded within the NHS, take somewhat for granted. Not only does the NHS indemnify competent practitioners, but many professionals also hold indemnity through their Royal Colleges. Those working outside the NHS need to ensure they are also covered if they and their clients are to be afforded similar protection. A word of warning here – as with most colleges, the RCN will only indemnify nurses for their own practice, when working with other nurses who are members of the RCN or when working with non-health care workers. They will not indemnify practice that relies upon multidisciplinary health care – with two exceptions: occupational health nurses and members of the RCN expert witness database. Alternative indemnity sources thus have to be found.

Governance

Governance is something that affects and is affected by all aspects of professional and business practice. The term 'governance' is a versatile one. It is used in government, large and small businesses, the media, the army, clinical practice and research. In essence, it is the set of arrangements or system by which the affairs of the organisation are ordered and monitored. ANPs will be familiar with the governance surrounding their existing roles. In developing alliances – strategic or otherwise – thinking outside of the box may be required. Governance is there to support us and protect our patients, clients and partners. Established entrepreneurs may work with service level agreements, contracts, partnership agreements and so on. In Vignette 7.1, Steve will be working to PCT governance, business governance and practice governance. This may include working to protocols and audit cycles. In Vignette 7.2, Claire will be mindful of hospital Trust governance requirements, referral protocols, governance around the use of telecoms and confidentiality, as well as her professional code of conduct in offering telephone advice to GPs, patients and carers. Vignette 7.3 requires Mary to ensure that research governance is followed, ethical principles are adhered to, contract requirements are fulfilled by all parties and that financial management is sound. These are just some examples of governance which can help us to maintain standards. Wallace's (2004) work can be used again here – what governance is in place that informs the project at hand? What else is needed, how do you access information to bridge the gap? What governance are your alliance partners guided by, what works and what does not?

Audit

It is commonly understood that audit of services is one way of maintaining standards. Clearly it is impossible here to present audit from the three vignettes discussed, although it is interesting to note that the change Steve has made was directly related to an audit which showed a discrepancy in service expectations. It might be reasonable to ask how much difference audit results make if the ensuing service development had to be made outwith the organisation.

It is also noted (Traynor *et al.* 2006) that there is little measurement and outcome literature around nurses and entrepreneurial work. Much of the available literature is in the form of narratives from nurses, often describing intrapreneurial activity. There is almost nothing relating to pain.

Advanced nursing practice and strategic alliances

ANPs exploring the possibilities of forming alliances with others will need to be able to identify their own competencies in a variety of areas. The ANP competencies currently suggested by the NMC will help in starting this process, but someone moving towards entrepreneurship may find that there are other areas in which they identify a need for competence. In particular, these may include business skills such as marketing, which are not part of the ANP framework. Help with these can be found in other publications, including in 'Nurse entrepreneurs: turning initiative into independence' (RCN, 2007).

The area of competence will also depend upon the project being undertaken, but will often overlap. For instance, the research-based vignette might be considered to need competencies identified from the area of 'professional role', such as using research to implement the role of the ANP, that calls for the ANP to function in the role of the researcher, or another that calls upon the ANP to provide leadership in many forms. It would also encompass aspects of managing and negotiating health care delivery systems, in particular the negotiating skills identified. But we suggest it also encompasses the clinical competencies – for how can one advise on the use of, or assess the adequacy of, a particular pain assessment tool if one does not already have the skills needed to use it and recognise its place in clinical practice.

The ANP competencies, particularly in the sections on leadership and managing and negotiating health care delivery systems, provide some challenges to those who are considering becoming more entrepreneurial or developing alliances. Being actively involved in a professional organisation is more than just paying an annual subscription. It demonstrates a commitment to an area, to colleagues and to the development of that specialty. It shows that the individual engages more widely with current issues and enables him or her to maintain an awareness of contemporary health policy in relation to the area of work. You may want to ask yourself how aware you are of current health policy in relation to pain management. What national reports that impact on the delivery of pain services have been published in the last 2 years?

The ANP standards also require the nurse to have current knowledge of their organisation and of the financing of the health service. It may be that in the chronic pain clinic, your manager discusses with the medical consultant the impact of the changing Healthcare Resource Group (HRG) definitions when looking at the financial forecasts. But if you are to achieve the standard required, you too should be able to have that conversation. A lack of financial acumen and you cannot complete Wallace's first area of knowing yourself and your organisation. Vignette 7.1 demonstrated not just an ability to put a finger on the gap in service provision, but also how responding to that gap needed skills of negotiation, financial discussion and advocating for patients to enable the service to be developed.

All three vignettes show nurses in pain management working at the level of the ANP and, in some cases, beyond that in their ability to use alliances as a strategy to improve patient outcome. Claire demonstrates not just clinical expertise (which is expected from a clinical nurse specialist) but also an ability to bring people together (patient, health care professionals and carers) to form an alliance which supports the patient. This is a development clearly called for in the ANP competencies. It is one which some years ago might have been undertaken by doctors, but the development of different roles in nursing has given us the opportunity to develop these alliances in a much more transparent fashion, using the latent leadership skills of senior clinical nurses.

This chapter has also shown how nurses can develop the competencies required for ANP status and, by using alliances as part of a strategy, move beyond intrapreneurship into entrepreneurship, thus encompassing and transforming those competencies.

Conclusions

By considering the three vignettes, which exemplify different aspects of pain service delivery, this chapter has shown how developing alliances is part of the role of the ANP. Beyond that it has also shown how using alliances can be part of a strategy in developing entrepreneurial skills, showing how the ANP (if he or she wants to) can emerge, evolve and establish themselves as entrepreneurs.

ANPs will have, or will be developing, the skills which will enable them to make alliances with others. As in Claire's case, frequently the skill to be built upon is that of referral, for in making an appropriate referral one has to properly assess the patient's need and who might best provide for that. Skills in knowing yourself and the world of the person to whom you refer will help to ensure a successful outcome. But to build an alliance there is a slight shift in focus, no longer is one asking for advice or an opinion; in an alliance you are suggesting that working together can build something bigger than both parties working alone.

ANPs themselves will benefit from working in new and exciting ways, by developing existing skills and learning new ones, by broadening their horizons and facilitating enhanced personal and professional fulfilment. Vignette 7.3 in particular demonstrated this as Mary explored ways in which her business broadened its horizons when working in an alliance with others.

The range of opportunities that exist in developing alliances is, as we have already stated, bound only by imagination. Nevertheless, ANPs need structure and guidance to move forward with intra- and entrepreneurship. Frameworks, such as Wallace's (2004), can provide a useful starting point in thinking about one's own skills and the area in which new ways of working could be explored. Networks, such as the Nurse Entrepreneurs Forum, offer support and ideas and lessen isolation. Working with others through alliances enables such opportunities to be grasped.

In the current world of health care it is not only service provision which is changing. Patient expectations are also increasing, and many pain practitioners feel a responsibility to ensure that pain services go beyond meeting basic needs to maximising care. ANPs bring their clinical, communication, leadership and entrepreneurial skills to these services. They have unique opportunities to innovate and maximise the quality and effectiveness of pain management services. Steve (Vignette 7.1) found that an alliance made outwith secondary care enabled him to provide a service which worked to provide the quality that patients had identified.

In the particular world of pain management perhaps the best alliances we can make daily are with our patients. However, entrepreneurial ANPs need to also think outside of the box and consider that developing alliances with people other than patients will bring benefits, which are not currently being realised.

Acknowledgements

The authors gratefully acknowledge the assistance given in writing this chapter from Paul Bibby, consultant nurse, Sherwood Forest Hospitals NHS Trust, and Karin Cannons, pain nurse specialist, Frimley Park Hospitals NHS Foundation Trust.

References

Adams, P.R., 2001. Making strategic alliances work in the healthcare industry. *International Journal of Medical Marketing*, 1, 252–265.
Arie, S., 2006. Can GPs compete with big business? *BMJ*, 332, 1172–1173.

Burrows, D., 2006. The art and science of independent practice – what is this nurse up to? *British Pain Society Newsletter*, Spring, 26–27.

Crombie, A., 2006. Nurse partnership for a nurse practitioner. *Primary Health Care*, 16(4), 14–16.

Duysters, G., de Man, A.-P., Wildeman, L., 1999. A network approach to alliance management. *European Management Journal*, 17(2), 182–187.

Hughes, F., Duke, J., Bamford, A., Moss, C., 2006. Enhancing nursing leadership through policy, politics and strategic alliances. *Nurse Leader*, 4(2), 24–27.

Kautz, J., 2008. Small business notes. Available at http://www.smallbusinessnotes.com/operating/leadership/strategicalliances.html [accessed 25 February 2009].

Kennedy, S.P., Bormann, B.J., 2006. Effective partnering of academic and physician scientists with the pharmaceutical drug development industry. *Experimental Biology and Medicine*, 231(11), 1690–1694.

RCN, 2007. Nurse entrepreneurs: turning initiative into independence. Available at http://www.rcn.org.uk/__data/assets/pdf_file/0018/115632/003215.pdf [accessed 25 February 2009].

Spekman, R.E., Isabella, L.A., MacAvoy, T.C., Forbes, T., 1996. Creating strategic alliances which endure. *Long Range Planning*, 29, 346–357.

Traynor, M., Davis, K., Drennan, V., Goodman, C., Humphrey, C., Locke, R., Mark, A., Murray, S., Banning, M., Peacock, R., 2006. *A Report to The National Co-Ordinating Centre for NHS Service Delivery and Organisation R&D (NCCSDO) of a Scoping Exercise on 'The Contribution of Nurse, Midwife and Health Visitor Entrepreneurs to Patient Choice'*. Available at http://www.entreprenurses.net/pubs/sdo.pdf [accessed 16 June 2008].

Wallace, R., 2004. Strategic Partnerships: An Entrepreneur's Guide to Joint Ventures and Alliances. Chicago: Dearborn Trade.

Useful resources

Business Link, www.businesslink.gov.uk

Chambers of Commerce – local contact details available via your local library

Federation of Small Businesses, Tel.: 0151 346 9000, www.fsb.org.uk

The Athena Network, 61 Ebury Road, Rickmansworth, Hertfordshire, WD3 1 BL, www.theathenanetwork.com

Everywoman, 17 Wootton Street, London, SE1 8TG, Tel: 0870 746 1800, www.everywoman.com

LinkedIn, www.linkedin.com

Chapter 8
An overview of advanced nursing practice in the development of pain clinics in primary care: new ways of working

Paul Bibby

Introduction

The issue

The role of the nurse consultant was introduced as part of the government's plans to modernise the NHS. My appointment as a consultant pain nurse in 2001 led me to review local pain services in order to improve their structure so that a more patient-focused model could be developed. Excessive waiting lists, inadequate resources due to service investment not matching increasing service demand, and an ageing population in an area that also suffers high unemployment had come together to create a significantly oversubscribed outpatient service that was unable to provide preventative or curative treatment. This is not just a local problem as the Chronic Pain Policy Coalition identifies:

> Chronic pain affects 7.8 million people of all ages in every parliamentary constituency of the UK. But two recent independent reports support a government commissioned survey that identified pain services in the UK as 'variable and patchy.' When poorly managed, conditions associated with pain can have a devastating impact on the quality of life of individuals and their families, with 25% of those diagnosed with chronic pain losing their jobs and in 22% of cases chronic pain also leads to depression. The failure to implement an effective prevention and treatment strategy for chronic pain not only imposes an unnecessary burden on patients, but also represents an inefficient allocation of time, money and professional expertise. This includes 4.6 million GP appointments per year that often end without resolution leading to further appointments and £3.8 billion a year spent on incapacity benefit payments to those diagnosed with chronic pain (http://www.paincoalition.org.uk/challenge.html).

Outline

In an attempt to address the problem I embarked upon a project that started with an informal audit of patient opinion, led onto a qualitative research study and a pilot community pain clinic. In the aftermath of the evaluation I applied my findings by forming a private pain company that provides services for the NHS under Practice Based Commissioning and Choose and Book, and also participated in the redesign of services provided by the NHS Trust where I am employed. This chapter provides the reader with an overview of this process and informs others who seek to advance their nursing practice in the management of chronic pain.

Background – an overview of the provision of pain services

The provision of chronic pain services in the NHS in the UK has been primarily anaesthetic-led (Charlton 2003). Historically the predominant model has been interventionist, with long-term management of this benign problem relying upon techniques such as epidurals, facet joint injections and other 'hi-tech' strategies (Charlton 2003). However, with the advent of evidence-based medicine, it became apparent that much of the clinical practice within a traditional pain clinic might be regarded as art rather than science (Dobson 2000). For example, take the case of two of the commonest interventions in a pain clinic, namely caudal epidurals and acupuncture. It is known that by inserting (acupuncture) needles into the skin the release of both serotonin and endorphins can be achieved. It is also understood that the effects of a steroid injection into the epidural space can have an impact upon some of the chemical activity thought to be responsible for the pain associated with sciatica. Clinical trials involving these techniques have failed to generate the evidence required to validate the application of the relevant biochemistry. Yet there is probably not a pain clinic in the NHS that is not oversubscribed with patients who rely upon caudal epidurals or acupuncture (or indeed both) in order to maintain any level of quality of life.

Historical practices, though, have been established and many patients as well as clinicians believe in the perceived efficacy of treatments and service models. Reliance upon these approaches to pain management has been applied across the NHS, with increasing and significant numbers of satisfied customers. The utilisation of medicines management, acupuncture, transcutaneous electrical nerve stimulation (TENS), patient education and clinical psychology has also been developed and integrated into pain clinic service models (Charlton 2003).

Despite this proliferation of service development, it has been shown that care provided in different regions of the country for people suffering from persistent pain is patchy and under-resourced (Dr Foster 2004), highlighting the variations in the provision of such specialist services. Service provision has been identified to range from as little as one consultant seeing a few hundred patients per year to significant multidisciplinary clinical teams with administrative infrastructure supporting caseloads of several thousands, resulting in ratios of about one clinician to only 70 patients. Such is the disparity.

Patient pathways into pain clinics have also evolved as a result of creeping service developments. Subsequently access to pain clinics usually occurs after considerable time and multiple general practitioner (GP) and hospital attendances. For example, many pain clinics can still report that up to 70% of their patients come from consultant-to-consultant referrals and that often these patients have been managed with physical therapies and medications under the supervision of secondary care for some years (Bibby 2006). This process fosters the psychosocial comorbidities that are associated with various chronic disease states, leading to a culture of dependency upon medical treatments. Over time increasing numbers of patients have come to rely upon various regular interventionist treatments because chronicity had become established some time prior to attending a pain clinic (Bibby 2006).

However, it cannot be ignored that desirable outcomes are achieved for substantial numbers of patients despite the presence of established chronicity, significant time delays in waiting for treatments and pathways that fail to direct a patient towards effective interventions. This gave me the idea that the provision of specialist pain management services earlier in the patient journey could lead to a reduction of chronicity and its associated psychosocial comorbidities and to an improved utilisation of the health care resource.

Developing the service

Identifying a need

My personal involvement with the idea of community pain clinics began with a simple audit of patient satisfaction. The audit consisted of randomly offering a questionnaire to patients attending a secondary care NHS pain clinic until 50 completed questionnaires had been collected (see Appendix 1). This audit identified that patients perceived that the treatments they were having from the pain clinic did work. However, there were two issues that were consistently raised by participants. Firstly, it was perceived by 80% of those patients that participated in the audit that had the service been available sooner after their pain problem became established (earlier in the patient pathway) then many of the psychosocial problems they had endured could have been avoided (e.g. loss of employment, depression requiring medication). The second issue was about access as many patients had to travel over 20 miles to attend this pain clinic, and having access to a clinic much closer to home was repeatedly raised in patient responses.

As a direct result of the findings of this audit I began investigating the subject further. Before I did anything, I needed to establish the actual patient journey as it occurs locally and attempt to extract from this any experiences which either assisted or exacerbated the management of chronic pain. After initial literature searches I found, as had previous authors (Smith *et al.* 1999), that there is useful disease-specific and interventionist-minded material available to help inform service design and clinical strategies. What was lacking was any evidence of what happens when the tools are applied within varying service models (Bibby 2006). I identified that a retrospective survey of the patient journey across the local health community using semistructured interviews could provide me with useful evidence as to what elements of, and how, service design were contributing to the development of, or assisting in, the management of chronicity. Regardless of whether my hypothesis was correct or not, this study would generate data that could inform service redesign so that a prospective study looking at a proposed model could be conducted. It was agreed that this study would be restricted to patients attending the pain clinic who were suffering with neck pain. It was considered that this subgroup provided a representative cohort of the various demographics that typically occur within our patient group at the pain clinic.

The study identified that following long periods of management by GPs, physiotherapists and orthopaedic consultants, these patients eventually found relief for their symptoms when being treated at the pain clinic with a combination of patient education, acupuncture and medicines management. Key to the study was that often patients had previously been treated with acupuncture, patient-centred pain management education and prescriptions of analgesics, but outside of the pain clinic environment and without success. It is entirely possible, therefore, that either the expertise of the clinical team within the pain clinic or the 'experience' of attending the pain clinic have an affect on the outcome of treatments. This provided me with a basis to provide these treatments in a pain clinic setting in primary care in an attempt to identify if any improvements could be achieved by offering the effective 'package of care' but earlier in the patient pathway. Further details of this research and service development are to be found in Bibby (2006).

It is important to point out that such concepts are in no way unique. Stannard and Johnson (2003) purport that the management of chronic pain belongs within the community setting for many reasons, including the need to educate the patient to take responsibility and control and to understand the patient's pain within the context of the family and society of which they are a part. However, most primary care organisations have no or little recommendations or budgets for the provision of chronic pain management within the community (Dr Foster 2004).

Rationale for change

The implications of this research, though limited, as this was a qualitative study, highlight a number of pertinent points (Bibby 2006). Firstly, once patients attended the pain clinic, they gained an improved understanding of their condition as a result of the specialist knowledge and understanding that pain specialists demonstrated. It is hypothesised that the effect of this rapport between patient and practitioner may have had an impact on the efficacy of subsequent treatments. Secondly, patients also recognised that if treatments such as acupuncture could work after such complex, ineffective and lengthy clinical pathways, then surely earlier access to effective treatments will achieve at least equal clinical outcomes, but without the burden on the patient, and therefore on society, of increasing chronicity and repeated hospital and GP attendances. This was raised in the audit by patients as well. Thirdly, it is evident that the combination of patient education and acupuncture can be delivered by a non-medical practitioner. Other aspects of ongoing patient care included medicines management and the use of TENS. This comprises an 'intervention set' that can be delivered by a nurse specialist, working within a community setting.

As identified by the Southampton Pain Service project 'Managing Pain Management' (Price & Parker 2006) there is a need to address key elements of service provision in order to optimise the potential for more clinical and cost–effective pain management (see Box 8.1). The award-winning project in Southampton was borne of repeated

Box 8.1 The Southampton Service.

- Demand management – making sure the right person gets seen in the right place at the right time
- Service redesign – structuring the service to permit a biopsychosocial approach
- Appropriate management of patient expectations
- Clear care pathways to take a person in and out of the service

Bulletin 36, p1830-2 The Royal College of Anaesthetists March 2006

crises emerging between commissioners and providers. But the development of pain clinics in primary care remains limited despite the high-profile resource produced by the Southampton project. As highlighted earlier, the subject is not a new one. In 1999, Smith *et al.* published a review article 'Chronic pain in primary care' in which the key issues that still pose a challenge to both commissioners and providers, as well as the actual clinicians themselves, are discussed. In particular is the discussion in this article about the need to move away from condition-specific treatment to the perception of chronic pain as an entity in itself, and so to approach its management in an entirely holistic manner. Furthermore, the development of a team of practitioners to work cohesively to meet the needs of this patient group is addressed. Price and Parker (2006) are equally insistent on the need for treating chronic pain using a multidisciplinary biopsychosocial approach, and while the understanding for the need to manage pain within the context in which it occurs has been discussed for several years (Stannard & Johnson 2003) Southampton represents the first formal attempt to redesign pain services through a chronic disease management approach.

Formulating a service model

It was important to establish if there was any evidence available that could direct the service model. Five studies were retained from searches in preparation to conduct this project. These were Thomsen *et al.* (2001), Karjalainen *et al.* (2003), Turner-Stokes *et al.* (2003), Temmink *et al.* (2000) and Horrocks *et al.* (2002).

Thomsen *et al.* (2001) conducted a systematic review of the economic effectiveness of multidisciplinary team (MDT) pain management for any subset of chronic pain and concluded that without the use of standard costing and outcome measurement methodology, it is not possible to identify evidence. Karjalainen *et al.* (2003) conducted a systematic review into the effectiveness of MDT approaches to rehabilitate those suffering with chronic neck and shoulder pain and concluded that a paucity of scientific evidence exists to suggest that MDT approaches are clinically effective. Turner-Stokes *et al.* (2003) continue with the theme that there is no advantage from the expense of an MDT. However, the intervention used in this study (cognitive behavioural therapy) was shown to be effective whether by individual therapy or MDT group therapy. Temmink *et al.* (2000) review the practice of implementing service redesign in which care is provided for people with chronic disease by the most appropriate professional at the lowest cost level. They also suggest that the inclusion of advanced nursing practice in such innovations is normally included in primary care-orientated countries, but that the influences on cost, quality and patients' preferences remain unclear. Horrocks *et al.* (2002) conducted a systematic review of studies to identify if nurse practitioners working in primary care can provide equivalent care to doctors. Statistical analysis of data from these papers showed that there was no difference in health outcomes. Although this suggests that the use of nurse-led clinics does not diminish quality of care over the use of a medical practitioner, it will be important to focus on the implications of longer consultations, as identified by Horrocks *et al.* (2002), in respect of economic evaluation of the service. There is quite simply nothing identified in these papers to suggest that a nurse-led service model should not be trialled.

Challenges

The added value of the nurse consultant role

I wanted to establish a nurse-led clinic for patients with chronic neck (and shoulder) pain within the community. I wanted this service to take referrals directly from GPs and I was eager to evaluate clinical effectiveness, cost-effectiveness and user satisfaction. I began to appreciate the uniqueness of the nurse consultant role and the opportunity it can afford the individual in post, as well as nursing as a whole. I had the opportunity to take a clinical lead on the strategic development of this service and the opportunity to influence this. Using my own research and learning epitomises for me the potential and personal fulfilment that can be realised from the nurse consultant role.

I was positioned between a number of significant stakeholders from primary and secondary care, creating a situation in which I had to coordinate a project that meant working across organisational boundaries; there seemed to be very little shared vision between the PCTs and secondary care, so it was not simply a case of going through the motions with others. I found that my nursing background helped me to continuously return agendas to a patient-centred focus when clinicians felt that traditional systems were being needlessly undermined. While my expert knowledge of pain management carried me when I was presenting the case for a service redesign, it was the process of managing change at this level, with no other champion for the cause that really was to be my opportunity for personal and professional expansion. I learned to trust myself in new and dynamic situations and it was this that raised my personal and professional expectations, so that when I began to realise that I was going to make very little progress in achieving my goals unless I did something radical, it meant that I needed the self-belief to do that radical act; and so the idea to form my own company and make that the vehicle for change was born.

Achieving cross-organisational agreement

A service level agreement needed to be formulated. I brought together key individuals from primary and secondary care in order to construct this project. I demonstrated, based on the work that I had done, the potential for improving patient services. I also made use of committees already in place that had been established to examine orthopaedic (related) services. Membership of these committees included secondary care service development managers, orthopaedic consultants, primary care-based physiotherapy managers, GP leads at PCT level and PCT commissioning managers. None of the medical pain consultants wished to be involved. However, being an NHS consultant myself meant that this did not equate to disarmament of my vision.

All representatives from primary care were proactively supportive, but there were issues for secondary care. In particular, there was the potential for undermining the trust's position as the provider of choice. However, the purpose of the nurse consultant is to lead the development of new services across the health community, with a particular emphasis upon patient-centred care and improved access. Because I was prepared to take ownership of the responsibility upon me as a nurse consultant, I was able to influence the key stakeholders. Subsequently I gained the support for a 6-month trial. Inclusion and exclusion criteria, as well as the scope of the service were defined (see Box 8.2–8.4), and all GPs informed and invited to participate. It was agreed that this service would also include TENS in order to ensure that a range of basic pain specialist nurse interventions were available. Treatment always included patient education about their condition, their current medication and lifestyle factors that can impact positively or negatively upon their pain. Acupuncture was always the preferred modality of intervention, but in cases where it had proved ineffective or was contraindicated (e.g. on warfarin therapy), TENS was applied. Alterations to medication were always carried out in consultation with the patients GP.

Box 8.2 Inclusion criteria.

- Registered with participating GP
- Adults (18 years +)
- Identifiable neck pain
- Absence of malignancy
- Absence of clear need for surgical intervention/assessment

Box 8.3 Exclusion criteria.

- Under 18 years of age
- Absence of identifiable neck pain
- Malignancy
- Requirement for surgical intervention/assessment
- Ongoing substance misuse

Box 8.4 Scope of the service.

- The service is available to all GPs within the participating PCT.
- This is NOT a diagnostic service.
- This service has referrals access to secondary care and clinical psychology.
- All patients are assessed by a specialist pain nurse, including
  - a detailed history,
  - a physical examination,
  - assessment for 'red flags',
  - assessment for 'yellow flags'.
- Treatment options will include
  - patient education,
  - medication review,
  - acupuncture,
  - TENS.

Evaluation

Clinical outcomes

All patients that were referred were asked to complete a Brief Pain Inventory (BPI) prior to any interventions. Patients were assessed and a treatment plan identified, or when appropriate referred back to their GP, or on to a secondary care pain clinic. If treatment was initiated, then the BPI was repeated within 1 week after completion of treatment. BPI scores were separated into two categories: pain scores and quality of life scores.

Eight GP practices participated in the pilot. From these a total of 20 patients were referred. Sixteen patients received effective treatments, showing at least 30% improvement in particular components of their BPI scores. Of the remaining four, two were immediately referred on to secondary care for a review by a consultant in pain medicine due to the complexity of their pain history, and two did not respond to the nurse-led treatments (i.e., they did not demonstrate at least a 30% improvement in BPI scores) and were subsequently referred on to secondary care for a review by a consultant in pain medicine.

Learning about service development from the experience

Each stakeholder could identify a number of potential benefits that this project offered. For example, the secondary care Acute Trust (where chronic pain services are traditionally provided) identified the possibility of being able to focus its activity on more complex case management, reduce waiting list pressures and look to the future of being in a position, as a foundation trust, to secure contracts to provide community-based services such as the one that could emerge as a result of this project. Primary care trusts identified the potential to transfer chronic disease management from secondary care, improve access to specialist services and reduce the frequency of unnecessary secondary care referrals.

This project can be defined as an innovation in health service delivery in that it meets the criteria set out by Greenhalgh *et al.* (2004). Being perceived as a new service and linked to the provision of existing pain management services, it is also discontinuous with the traditional model of a medically led service. Having emerged entirely from nursing audit, nursing research and reflection upon practice, it exemplifies the unique contribution that the nurse consultant can make to patient care. Furthermore, it is directed at improving outcomes, efficiency, cost-effectiveness and user experience.

Diffusion of innovation theory

In that this project is an innovation, diffusion of innovation theory provides a basis for a critique of the process. Diffusion of innovation theory suggests that the process of diffusion is that by which a new idea is spread from the source of invention or creation to where it will be utilised (Rogers 1983). Although the process of developing the detail of the project and agreeing the manner in which it would be diffused through a cross-organisational mesh was achieved with relative ease, it became inherently clear within the first 6 weeks of implementation that significant numbers of referrals were not being made. This has remained the key point for consideration in reviewing the implementation process. In the first instance, despite the efforts of PCT personnel, many GPs did not actually know of the service. Secondly, some GPs expected a pain service to be led by a medical consultant and so were reluctant to try this new approach.

The description of innovation development based on Rosenau (1998, p. 25, Figure 3) who describes a process of filters that sifts out innovations or projects in stages. It helps to explain why this problem occurred.

Early stage filters

Projects that do not match with organisations long-term goals and those that can be delivered after an analysis of near-term resources/priorities will be sidelined fairly quickly. This project appealed to the long-term health sector targets for chronic disease management and transferring of services from secondary to primary care, for example 'a patient-led NHS' (DH 2005). Furthermore, it required more than an analysis of resources and priorities. So it survived to be implemented.

Faulty filtering

However, this project was developed through what might be described as a faulty filter system. If there has been one error in the implementation process, it was to not consult with all GPs *directly*. An assumption was made that GP representation at PCT level was adequate. However, more involved negotiation with GPs could have ensured that the following was embedded within the project design and implementation process:

(1)   GPs would have known about the service.
(2)   GPs would have influenced the service design.

(3)   GPs would have felt ownership of the service.
(4)   GPs who wanted access to medical staff could have influenced a strategy for such a provision within the service design.

Adoption process

Had the diffusion of this innovation been delivered via an effective filter system, that had reflected the pivotal importance of direct consultation with GPs, it would have led to 'the adoption process', a concept also discussed by Rogers (1983). Having gained awareness of the innovation by virtue of direct approaches by the project management team, GPs would have had the opportunity to gain interest by virtue of learning more through the consultation process. Subsequent referrals to the service would have provided an opportunity for them to evaluate and then progress to the trial stage during which the innovation would have become an established point for referral. This would then have secured the adoption of the model for longer term commissioning.

Reflection

Successful project management depends upon effective planning. The problem in this case is not, for example, whether or not a force field analysis was undertaken, but rather if the insight that existed regarded what the forces to be analysed actually were. Organisational culture and how organisations interact with one another can be the difference between a particular project design being a success or not (Handy 1993). It is therefore paramount that an understanding exists not only of how PCTs and Secondary Care Trusts interact generally, but also how the particular Trusts involved interact specifically with one another. Furthermore, an understanding of how other stakeholders (i.e. GPs) interact with (in) these organisations must be clear. It is possible that a keener awareness of the politics that exist between GPs (who see themselves as the 'gatekeepers' of health care provision) and PCTs (who have been the Department of Health's ambassadors of health care commissioning), particularly during a time when practice-based commissioning is being introduced, may have inspired a more direct involvement of GPs opinions and preferences for this project.

Pettigrew and Whipp (1991) describe an environment for effective change in which a number of contexts are receptive to a proposed innovation. Contexts, such as environmental pressures, organisational culture, coherence and quality of policy, organisational goals, leaders of change and change/locale, did not provide stumbling blocks and even expedited the process. However, the cooperation between GPs and PCTs, and the nature of this managerial–clinical relationship proved to be a costly oversight.

Following an interim appraisal I approached GP practices and consulted directly about the service. It was clear from this that as the evidence suggests, GPs felt more involved and able to stake their claim in this project. Subsequently, referral numbers increased to more acceptable levels.

Rosenau (1998) describes that project management can be inherently frustrating due to the many directions that various organisations might appear to (and probably actually will) be heading. Such frustrations are created by the simple fact that the project manager does not have control over the behaviour of individuals or organisations. Such behaviour is the perfectly natural and appropriate way for communities of people to act

(Handy 1993). So it can be understood that it is not the behaviour of the communities of people, be they GPs, the project team or a particular NHS trust, that has been the problem here. A more thorough preparation, achieved by analysing the situation more closely could have identified the potential for a breakdown in communication and progression of the project unless GPs were centred in the consultation process. Change is influenced by 'historical, cultural, economic and political factors' (Iles & Sutherland 2001) and to overlook key political factors can only have undermined the process.

Evaluation – theory and process

The focus of evaluation of this project is rooted in an original piece of research conducted locally (Bibby 2006). This study identified that there was potential to improve the management of chronic neck pain by placing an 'intervention' at the beginning of the patient journey, which has traditionally been provided after some years of chronicity. This 'intervention' combines medicines management by a specialist practitioner, patient education and acupuncture.

In identifying how to evaluate this project, consideration was given not only to clinical outcomes, but also the need to examine the changes to the patient pathway, particularly access and the impact of early intervention, as well as various details related to cost-effectiveness. The number of other variables that could contribute to any identified changes in outcomes also needs to be tracked and monitored in order to provide a comprehensive assessment.

As previously mentioned a similar, but much larger, project had previously been conducted in Southampton, attracting the McKinsey Award for the best innovation in health care leadership at the Medical Futures Innovation Awards on 3 November 2005 (British Pain Society 2006). From that project a package of implementation and evaluation tools to assist clinical teams in developing primary care-based pain services had been produced. This package provided a resource that assisted in the production a comprehensive evaluation of this project against the aims and objectives outlined in Box 8.5.

Box 8.5 Aims and objectives of the evaluation process.

Aims
- Evaluate the clinical benefits of a chronic neck pain service where there is a significant primary-care-based intervention.
- Evaluate the processes produced by setting up a primary care based chronic neck pain clinic.

Objectives
- Evaluate the clinical outcomes achieved by providing an intervention (specialist medicines management, patient education and acupuncture) for chronic neck pain in a primary care setting.
- Evaluate access and waiting list management achieved by this primary-care-based service.
- Evaluate user satisfaction with the primary-care-based service.
- Evaluate the cost effectiveness of the primary-care-based service.

Evaluation can be described as either a formative or summative process (Bowling 2002). If the focus of the evaluation is to determine how to improve or develop an already established service, then it might normally be described as formative. However, a summative evaluation would be conducted in order to identify whether or not a service is worth continuing with. This project will inform commissioning bodies if adding this model alongside existing services will lead to improvement or not for patients and service providers, and to this effect one might assume that a formative evaluation is to be conducted. However, the crux is to identify whether or not this new initiative should be commissioned long term, or if service development should be taken in another direction. To this effect a summative evaluation should be conducted, though this might be viewed as part of a formative evaluation of the chronic pain service per se.

Øvretveit (1998) describes four types of evaluation, formative, process, implementation and outcome. It should be said at this stage that these four evaluation spheres do overlap, and so, as this discussion progresses, it is inevitable that any one-evaluation sphere could be applied differently. He views formative evaluation as an assessment about the direction that things are going in, and might be conducted as an interim review. This is not dissimilar to an evaluation of the implementation process, as previously described, in which it was identified that uptake of the service by GPs had been negatively affected by the manner in which they had (not) been consulted when developing service agreements. The term implementation evaluation focuses more directly on what factors have assisted or hindered the extent to which the project worked. Similarly, this remains closer to the review of the actual implementation process, giving insight into the way the service was developed.

In order to show if there are benefits to a new service structure, it is essential to evaluate processes (see Box 8.5). To ask how it's users are experiencing this service development gives insight into the quality of its processes. This is an important component of evaluating the primary care-based neck pain clinics, as without this evidence, it is difficult to make a judgement about other outcomes. For example, if patients are not gaining any significant improvement other than can be expected with a traditional model, is this because early intervention is of no value for this subgroup, or alternatively does the process evaluation demonstrate that a large proportion of those referred actually already had significant chronicity? Furthermore, it might then be shown that even if this is so, it is (or is not) cost-effective to redesign the service, even though no clinical improvement would be achieved.

Outcome evaluation can provide an analysis of what has been achieved in terms of actual clinical effect. This is vital as without it there is no evidence that the proposed intervention is of value to patients suffering with chronic neck pain. It is not unfeasible to anticipate either that increased outcome can be achieved due to earlier intervention or that less effectiveness is achieved because the outcomes associated with this intervention in the traditional model had relied upon other interventions first, which have now been removed.

Below is an appraisal of the types of tools that can be used in order to provide a comprehensive project evaluation.

Satisfaction questionnaires

User satisfaction needs to focus on GP and patient appraisal of detailed components of the care pathway, ensuring that a clear view of how those processes might have helped or hindered the effectiveness of the service, the value placed on it by users and why. The necessity of evaluating systems, although clearly discussed by various authors (Øvretveit 1998), can easily be overlooked. If health care organisations are to improve their ability to provide services that meet the needs of their target audience, then process evaluation must be viewed as essential feedback about the extent to which service design is correct (Kotler & Clarke 1987). If users do not like a service design, they will seek other avenues to access the clinical intervention, especially in this current era of patient choice (DH 2005).

Although there is a wealth of questionnaires available for this kind of appraisal, local NHS evaluation audit and research departments are suitably qualified and skilled to assess them.

Clinical outcomes questionnaires

A popular clinical outcomes tool in chronic pain management is the BPI Short Form (Cleeland & Ryan 1994). Although originally developed for use in cancer pain management, Tan *et al.* (2004) conducted a study to evaluate the validity of this tool for use in chronic non-malignant pain, finding that not only is this tool a valid instrument, but it assesses related and distinct dimensions. What is important from a clinical point of view is that Tan *et al.* (2004) have provided evidence to assure the practitioner that correlations can be relied upon as genuinely being related to one another.

This tool provides a comprehensive overview of the patients' pain scores and the impact of pain on selected aspects of daily living. By measuring both sensory and reactive dimensions of the pain experience, it provides an assessment of a person's pain intensity and the extent to which this is interfering with their daily life. This is important, as many people will improve their function to the point at which pain is a problem for them. In such cases, the pain score may not alter very much, while those scores that reflect the impact of pain upon daily living reduce significantly. By repeating completions of the forms on a routine basis means that a picture not unlike an observation chart will emerge. This can help influence clinical management as well as validate it.

More detailed assessments are sometimes used in clinical practice (Newton-John 2003), but the intellectual ability of patients varies and a number may be significantly depressed, or be distracted by anxiety, and so lack the motivation to complete lengthy and complex forms. However, at the other end of this scale it would be undermining of the process to use other validated assessment tools such as 'The Duke Health Profile' (Wu *et al.* 2002) that might be considered too simplified, resulting in less clear outcome data.

Conclusions

It is not uncommon for nurses to feel that despite their great ideas, they are unable to take them forward. This can be for various reasons; not least of all is the codependency that is inherent within the profession (Bibby 2006). The opportunity for nursing and nurses is to realise that as the principles of 'adult' become increasingly inherent to us, so it will become equally likely that the 'child' behaviour displayed by our profession in the past will become displaced and so less likely to invoke a 'parent' response from others (Bibby 2005). More importantly, when others feel the need to behave in 'parent', the position of 'adult' disarms their behaviour (Harris 1973). Professional roles such as nurse consultant reflect the evolving character that has is now as inherent as our legacy of the past. With it comes the opportunity to drive forward our vision for our patients. This project has been like a catalyst that catapulted me into an entrepreneurial adventure, resulting in the formation of my own health care company and the creation of my own community pain services – not something I expected to achieve when I entered nursing.

A local GP, one of the co-authors of the article by Stannard and Johnson (2003), joined me in forming the company (Pain Management Solutions Ltd). Since that time the company has become an established provider of community pain services in South Yorkshire and Nottinghamshire, demonstrating that while the whole MDT is essential, many patients can safely access a pain service without being seen by the medical consultant. Furthermore, we have started to show how earlier access does help to reduce the impact of chronicity. Such is our success that we have recently been awarded a central contract by the Department of Health and will be appearing on the Free Choice Network from April 2009. From one simple audit, and thanks to the opportunities that are now afforded to nurses through our profession, I find myself in the driving seat of a major entrepreneurial adventure.

Appendix 1: Pain clinic audit

Patient Questionnaire

Thank you for agreeing to participate in this audit. As the information you provide is in confidence we do not require any personal details from you on this form. Simply complete it, enclose it within the envelope provided and give it to the receptionist on leaving.

1. What do you value most about the pain clinic?
2. What changes would you make to the way we deliver this service?
3. What would you like to have been different about the way your pain was managed prior to attending the pain clinic?

References

Bibby, P., 2005. Alcoholism and addiction: the management of spiritual pain in the clinical environment. In Schofield, P. (ed.), *Beyond Pain*. London: Whurr.

Bibby, P., 2006. The management of chronic neck pain – a retrospective survey of the patient journey using in-depth semi-structured interviews. *Journal of Orthopaedic Nursing*, 10, 25–32.

Bowling, A., 2002. *Research Methods in Health: Investigating Health and Health Services*, 3rd edn. Buckingham: OUP.

British Pain Society, 2006. Innovative restructuring of Pain Services attracts award. *British Pain Society Spring Newsletter*, 20–21.

Charlton, E.J., 2003. Organisation and facilities for chronic pain clinics: a UK perspective. In Jensen, T., Wilson, P., Watson, P., Haythornthwaite, J.A. (eds), *Clinical Pain Management: Chronic Pain*, pp. 155–162. London: Arnold.

Cleeland, C.S., Ryan, K.M., 1994. Pain assessment: global use of the Brief Pain Inventory. *Annals of Academic Medicine*, 23(2), 129–138.

DH, 2005. Creating a patient-led NHS: delivering the NHS improvement plan. Available at http://www.dh.gov.uk/PublicationsAndStatistics/Publications/PublicationsPolicyAnd-Guidance/PublicationsPolicyAndGuidanceArticle/fs/en?CONTENT_ID=4106506&chk=ftV6vA [accessed 3 March 2009].

Dobson, F., 2000. The art of pain management. *Professional Nurse*, 15(12), 786–790.

Dr Foster of Long-Term Medical Conditions Alliance (LMCA) UPA, 2004. *Adult Chronic Pain Management Services in the UK*. London: Dr Foster.

Greenhalgh, T., Robert, G., MacFarlane, F., Bate, P., Kyriakidou, O., 2004. Diffusion of innovations in service organisations: systematic review and recommendations. *The Milbank Quarterly*, 82(4), 581–629.

Handy, C., 1993. *Understanding Organisations*, 4th edn. London: Penguin.

Harris, T.A., 1973. *I'm OK – You're OK*, 3rd edn. London: Pan.

Horrocks, S., Anderson, E., Salisbury, C., 2002. Systematic review of whether nurse practitioners working in primary care can provide equivalent care to doctors. *BMJ*, 324, 819–823.

Iles, V., Sutherland, K., 2001. *Organisational Change: A Review for Health Care Managers, Professionals and Researchers*. London: National Coordinating Centre for NHS Service Delivery and Organisation.

Karjalainen, K.A., Malmivaara, A., van Tulder, M.W., Rione, R., Jauhiainen, M., Hurri, H., Koes, B.W., 2003. Multidisciplinary biopsychosocial rehabilitation for neck and shoulder pain among working age adults. *The Cochrane Database of Systematic Reviews*, Issue 2, Art No.: CD002194.

Kotler, P., Clarke, R.N., 1987. *Marketing for Health Care Organisations*, Chapter 10. New Jersey: Prentice-Hall.

Newton-John, T.R.O., 2003. Psychological effects of chronic pain and their assessment in adults. In Jensen, T.S., Wilson, P.R., Rice, A.S.C. (eds), *Clinical Pain Management: Chronic Pain*, Chapter 7. London: Arnold.

Øvretveit, J., 1998. *Reviews: Evaluating Health Interventions*. Buckingham: OUP.

Pettigrew, A., Whipp, R., 1991. *Managing Change for Competitive Success*. Oxford: Blackwell.

Price, C., Parker, D., 2006. *Managing Pain Management*, Bulletin 36, pp. 1830–1832. RCA.

Rogers, E., 1983. *Diffusion of Innovation*. New York: Free Press.

Rosenau, M.D., 1998. *Successful Project Management: A Step-by-Step Approach with Practical Examples*, 3rd edn. New York: Wiley.

Smith, B.H., Hoptonm, J.L., Chambers, A.W., 1999. Chronic pain in primary care. *Family Practice*, 16(5), 475–482.

Stannard, C., Johnson, M., 2003. Chronic pain management – can we do better? An interview-based survey in primary care. *Current Medical Research and Opinion*, 19(8), 703–706.

Tan, G., Jensen, M.P., Thornby, J.I., Shanti, B.F., 2004. Validation of the Brief Pain Inventory for chronic non-malignant pain. *Pain*, 5(2), 33–37.

Temmink, D., Francke, A.L., Hutten, J.B.F., Van Der Zee, J., Abu-Saad, H.H., 2000. Innovations in the nursing care of the chronically ill: a literature review from an international perspective. *Journal of Advanced Nursing*, 31(6), 1449–1458.

Thomsen, A.B., Sørensen, J., Sjøgren, P., Eriksen, J., 2001. Economic evaluation of multidisciplinary pain management in chronic pain patients: a qualitative systematic review. *Journal of Pain and Symptom Management*, 22(2), 688–698.

Turner-Stokes, L., Erkeller-Yuksel, F., Miles, A., Pincus, T., Shipley, M., Pearce, S., 2003. Outpatient cognitive behavioural pain management programs: a randomised comparison of a group-based multidisciplinary versus an individual therapy model. *Archives of Physical Medicine and Rehabilitation*, 84(6), 781–788.

Wu, L.R., Parkerson, G.R., Doraiswamy, P.M., 2002. Health perception, pain, and disability as correlates of anxiety and depression symptoms in primary care patients. *Journal of American Board of Family Practitioners*, 15, 183–190.

Chapter 9
Development of nurse-led pain management programmes: meeting a community need

Dee Burrows

Introduction

This chapter considers the development and nurse-led leadership of a multidisciplinary team in developing a pain management programme (PMP) and associated services in the independent sector. The challenges faced in implementing, growing and continuing to develop the service are considered. Approaches to maintaining standards, evaluation and audit – from the perspective of practitioners, patients and referrers – are discussed. The advanced nursing contribution will be summarised and deliberated further in relation to the wider opportunities.

One in seven of the UK population experiences chronic pain; there is an adult with pain in every third household; 49% of adults with chronic pain have had to take time off work and around a third has to give up work. Chronic pain is the second most common reason, after poor mental health, for being on incapacity benefit. Just under half of adults with chronic pain are depressed (Chronic Pain Policy Coalition 2007). Chronic pain impacts upon the individual and their ability to manage home, work and leisure activities; upon the family – in altered roles, relationships, finances, workloads and health; and upon society in increased health and social care costs and decreased expertise and contribution to the economy. Of course many people with chronic pain lead fulfilling lives, having learnt how to manage their pain.

There are a number of approaches to learning and implementing pain management strategies. This chapter confines itself to PMPs.

The first PMPs were developed in the early 1970s in Seattle, USA. Based on operant conditioning, they focused upon altering pain behaviours (Fordyce *et al.* 1973). Ten years later, Turk *et al.* (1983) cognitive behavioural therapy (CBT) into pain management. CBT essentially aims to change the way people think by challenging their beliefs about pain and thereby influencing behaviour. Until recently, CBT has been the predominant therapeutic approach used with people attending PMPs. The first UK outpatient programme was developed at the Walton Centre in 1983 and the first inpatient programme at St Thomas Hospital in 1988. Currently, McCracken and colleagues at the Bath Pain Management Unit are developing a *third-wave* approach (to distinguish from operant conditioning and CBT). Contextual cognitive behavioral therapy (CCBT) integrates acceptance and commitment therapy

(ACT) with mindfulness-based treatments (Vowles & McCraken 2008). According to Wicksell *et al.* (2009) ACT promotes acceptance rather than avoidance of something that cannot be changed and favours of engagement in meaningful activity despite pain.

As anyone working on PMPs will testify, there is a tendency to see this intervention as an 'end-of-the-line' treatment. Yet the stated aims of PMPs are to enhance self-management and rehabilitation – thus normalising, as far as possible, the pain experience and its impact and facilitating empowerment to change. In the mid-1990s there was increasing emphasis upon the importance of early intervention in both acute and chronic health care. The perceived rationale was that the earlier one intervened the quicker the recovery, the sooner people could return to their life roles at home, work and in leisure, the less the chronicity. Minimal evidence existed for this view – but it seemed to 'make sense'. At this time (as well as contributing to an NHS PMP) I was head of department at a university. She knew only to well the drive to incorporate innovation in the community into under and postgraduate curricula – yet understanding 'how' this might be done and finding practice examples was an entirely different matter.

Pain services are one aspect of health care that fit well in primary care. Pain is one of the top three reasons for people to visit their GPs and with few exceptions (such as the insertion of spinal cord stimulators) treatments can be carried out in the community. Furthermore work by, for example, Green (2006), on the management of musculoskeletal disorders in the workplace, has begun to indicate that early intervention has an evidence base of benefit for the patient, their family and the economy. Indeed, early access to treatment is one of the Chronic Pain Policy Coalition's (2007) five manifesto points. Early access is likely to be found more readily in community settings.

The community in this chapter are people with pain – not patients. People have families, friends, acquaintances and colleagues. People dip in and out of services – whether it be a post-office or primary care service. They seek a service for a specified need. In pain management the need can impact on many aspects of personal, family and working lives. Secondly, the community is the practitioners who deliver PMPs, working with individuals and their families. Pain management has historically been led by anaesthetists (Main & Spanswick 2000). The British Pain Society's (2007) 'Recommended guidelines for pain management programmes for adults' advises that PMPs 'should not be delivered without input from a medically qualified person' (p. 18). Other core staff include clinical psychologists and physiotherapists. The guidelines add that practitioners, such as occupational therapists (OTs), nurses and pharmacists, 'have skills which are extremely useful for the delivery of PMPs and may bring added value' (p. 19).

Some years ago, I began to contribute to a local NHS PMP that had been set up in 1996 by two OTs. It was this PMP that provided the grounding to develop skills in facilitating PMP delivery and in understanding PMP systems and processes. This understanding was later used to develop the nurse-led primary care-based PMP to which the chapter refers. Advanced nurse practitioners (ANPs) must seek opportunities and seize initiatives. With increasing nurse involvement and expertise in pain management and nurse prescribing, it is timely for nurses to consider their potential for bringing their 'added value' to developing and leading PMPs.

Developing the service

Building the team

The NHS PMP team referred to in the introduction had, for some time, been considering the idea of developing an independent early intervention service in primary care. With the knowledge and support of the trust's medical director, the NHS Programme's clinical psychologist set up a series of evening meetings. The ideas and motivation were sound; the commitment – with full time jobs and family responsibilities – was sadly unrealistic. The medical director expressed his regret, the Psychologist retired and life continued.

A couple of years later, I left university employment and with the encouragement of family, friends and the medical director, set up PainConsultants – an independent health care provider that specialises in 'working with people to reduce the impact of pain'. We achieve this through clinical services, training and education, research, consultancy and a small product division.

I am a practitioner, consultant nurse, the major shareholder and also the managing director. The first 3 months were spent considering the nature of the organisation and getting the team together. A consultant nurse and previous colleague came on board to share leadership of the training and education. A colleague of this nurse, who I had supervised when he and the nurse had undertaken a study on gender and pain, agreed to share leadership of the research. Both have an interest in the impact of pain on adult family carers, meaning that we could look at developing a research programme as well as potentially undertaking contract research. The OTs and physiotherapist from the NHS programme were keen to join the clinical services and together with a consultant psychologist, started to discuss how we might move forward with the ideas mooted 2 years previously. We also approached a service user consultant to join the clinical team. This individual had considerable personal experience of acute and chronic nociceptive and neuropathic pain, as well as the wider context of the NHS. Many other people assisted in the development, whether clinical, business or marketing, they have all helped to shape the organisation.

The clinical psychologist was new to the practitioner team. At our first meeting the previous development ideas were shared and those for the future discussed. Borrill and West (2002) suggest that effective teams are ones who have clarity about and commitment to their objectives, involve all participants fully, focus on quality through regular analysis and feedback on team performance, and who support creativity and innovation. We spent time becoming a team, getting to know each other better as people and as practitioners. Values were shared, frameworks introduced, debate enabled, critique given and taken. My role involved preparing agendas, chairing the meetings, typing and circulating minutes, resourcing materials, developing the infrastructure to support programme development and delivery, researching and drafting the protocols, reading and networking. It was an immense undertaking.

Table 9.1   Inclusion and exclusion criteria

Elements that identify suitability	Elements that indicate further investigation or onward referral
Pain of 6 weeks or more	Assessed to have possible red flags[a]
Medically examined as suitable for a pain management programme	Assessed to have severe depression, alcoholism or dependency on illegal drugs
Assessed as suitable by a team member	Medical morbidity or planned treatments, which might prevent participation in the full programme
Able to access the programme and its materials	
Payment option in place	Assessed as unsuitable for a group programme
Signed consent and commitment contract	

[a]Red flags denote high risk. In pain management if someone is regarded as having a potential red flag, it is indicative of possible serious spinal pathology.

Designing the programme – screening

As a team we were clear that we wanted to focus on early intervention in a primary care setting, but knew we needed to write the programme from scratch. Given the teams experience in delivering PMPs and the availability of national (British Pain Society 2007) and international guidance, it took a considerable time to agree the wording and order of the programme aims. The debate was influenced by the fact that we wanted to ensure we had a focus on work – whether paid, voluntary or in the home for those who were parents or home managers. Our aims can be found at www.painconsultants.co.uk. One of our first considerations was to agree the admission and exclusion criteria (see Table 9.1).

A simple referral form was designed which enables suitability for assessment to be determined within a telephone appointment with the prospective participant or referrer. This practice has subsequently influenced the screening process for the NHS programme, which is now also completed by telephone taking approximately 15 minutes.

Mindful that we do not have the direct involvement of a medical practitioner within the core PMP clinical team, we had to consider how we would screen prospective participants as medically suitable. The referral form allows us to record whether red flags (see Appendix 1) have been assessed for prior to telephone screening. However, we were all in agreement that we needed to accept self-referrals if we were to try to provide early access and would also need to take referrals from practitioners who might be less well informed of red flags than perhaps we are ourselves. Our approach to this challenge is discussed later in the chapter.

Telephone screening also enables us to record whether or not the individual is depressed, but not the level of depression which also constitute the 'yellow flags' (see Appendix 1). This has to be undertaken as part of the assessment process. Our clinical psychologist has responsibility for further investigation of individuals found to have severe depression. The policy for those with evidence of dependency on alcoholism or illegal drugs is to advise individuals to seek an urgent appointment with their GP or referrer. In cases where the individual is deemed to be 'at risk', we will telephone the clinician and forward an urgent follow-up letter. Template letters were drafted to ensure the process could be managed with due speed.

Designing the programme – assessment

Considerable time was spent discussing our assessment approach. The psychologist led the debate and provided the resources whilst I collated the decisions and developed the surrounding materials, as well as developing our medication questionnaire, and the physiotherapist developed a physical activity profile. Our standardised questionnaire pack incorporates measures of cognitive coping, pain, anxiety, depression, functional activity, fear avoidance, physical activity, medication and readiness for learning pain management strategies. Thus, the different biopsychosocial elements of pain are addressed via:

- Pain Coping Strategy Questionnaire (PCSQ; Rosential & Keefe 1983)
- Short-Form McGill Pain Questionnaire (SF-MPQ; Melzack 1987)
- Hospital Anxiety and Depression Scale (HADS; Zigmond & Snaith 1983)
- Beck's Depression Inventory II (BDI-II; Beck *et al.* 1996)
- Sickness Impact Profile (SIP; Gilson *et al.* 1975)
- Non Veterans Pain Outcome Questionnaire (Non-VA POQ; VA National Pain Outcomes Workgroup 2003)
- PainConsultants Physical Activity Profile (Deacon 2005)
- PainConsultants Medication Questionnaire (Burrows *et al.* 2005)
- Readiness for Change Questionnaire
- Record of goals

From the start we envisaged that we would take participants from outside of our immediate local area. As we wanted to value the person within their own context, rather than ours, we did not want them to come to us for assessment. We determined that we would either go to them assessing in their home/place of work or find an alternate way to assess. Clearly the whole team cannot travel to each potential participant. I travel on behalf of the core team and we have developed a team of associate practitioners around the country – other independent, individual practitioners in private practice and NHS practitioners seeking extra work. In addition, we investigated the pros and cons of telemedicine and other forms of technology.

The questionnaire pack is posted or emailed, according to the potential participant's preference, returned, scored, and the results are recorded in the individual's notes by consultant nurses. The full multidisciplinary team is available for consultation. The potential participant is then assessed face to face or via the telephone. The assessment form was designed by the team as a whole and allows the assessing practitioner to represent the different multidisciplinary perspectives. The only challenge for telephone assessments is that it is not possible to undertake either physical or functional assessments. As our confidence has grown, we have become able to discern when telephone assessments are or are not suitable. For instance, if the person has been seen by a medical consultant who has recommended a PMP, we are more likely to undertake a telephone assessment. Conversely, if from the referral information we are unclear about whether the person would best be helped by a PMP or one of our 1:1 pain education programmes (PEPs), we are more likely to undertake a face-to-face assessment.

Once the assessment form is completed, we provide feedback on the questionnaire results, discuss treatment options and goals and address any final questions. An assessment report is compiled in consultation with the multidisciplinary team as required, treatment recommendations are included and costed, and the report is sent to the referrer and potential participant. Responsibility for costing and referrer liaison lies with the consultant nurses. The process that was envisaged has had its glitches, but in essence has worked well.

Designing the programme – delivery

The CBT model introduced by the clinical psychologist enabled us to learn and develop as a team. Each of us had responsibility for writing certain group sessions and for tracking a theme through all the sessions. Having checked that physical sensations were addressed throughout, the psychologist focused on thoughts and feelings, the physiotherapist on behavioural aspects and the OT on environmental context and work. The service user consultant critiqued all handouts for ease of understanding. A programme manual and power point presentations were compiled and a participant handbook produced. Handbooks are sent out in advance and contain pre-course reading and written exercises introducing the individual to the philosophy of pain management, goal setting and the concepts of relaxation and exercise.

Initially, the programme was designed as an outpatient programme, one evening a week for 8 weeks supported by course work for the participant to undertake at home, work and in leisure. As is discussed further in the next section, demand and a change in referral routes led us to develop a programme for people with longer term pain and replace our outpatient programme with a residential one. The residential programme offers group sessions and individual appointments in Weeks 1 and 3, with participants testing their new skills in their own environments during Week 2 supported by telephone reviews with the consultant nurses and the 'course work partnership' system. This system provides each participant with a participant partner between and during sessions. Group sessions include:

- What is pain and pain management?
- Understanding, challenging and managing thoughts and feelings;
- Goal setting;
- Body dynamics, stretch and exercise;
- Managing activities and pacing at home and in the work place;
- Managing medication, stress, sleep and set backs;
- Problem solving at home and work;
- Carers' and employers needs.

In addition, each participant now has two individual appointments with both the physiotherapist and the OT, a medication review with a nurse if applicable, one to two appointments with the psychologist if required and two sessions with a key worker who is generally one of the nurses.

In developing the programme we needed to find a suitable venue. There is a private hospital within easy distance of our office. However, we wanted our programme to be located within a community, rather than health care setting. The two local village halls did not offer the type of environment we were looking for. We wanted somewhere that our participants felt valued and respected as people, rather than patients. Three of us visited and talked to two conference centres, both of which provide accommodation. The one we chose is set on the edge of the village and is a favourite venue for local weddings. It is within relatively easy distance of shops, a museum and open countryside (depending upon one's walking tolerance). Residence rooms are en suite and there are two rooms with facilities for wheelchair users. The venue staff are unfailingly flexible and accommodating of our participants' needs. Once we had the venue, we then needed to purchase books, CDs, pillows, mats and all the other equipment usually drawn upon in delivering PMPs.

Designing the programme – ongoing support and evaluation of progress

Formal reviews are undertaken 2 weeks after the residential stage has concluded and three monthly thereafter to the end of the year. The questionnaire pack is reapplied, followed by feedback of the results, discussion of progress and identification of goals for the coming 3 months. Interim reports are written for the participant, their GP and referrer. This process is undertaken by the consultant nurses.

In developing the PMP, the team felt that we could add value by offering participants 'ongoing support' to maximise internalisation of strategies and goal achievement. This element has become more important as we have developed the residential programme. The NHS PMPs, which the team has contributed to, have not historically been resourced to offer follow-up and we thus had no specific experience to draw upon. Nevertheless, the work put in during the development stage has stood us in good stead and we are now increasingly aware of the resources we can draw upon and indeed the nature of support we can offer. Again the consultant nurses hold the responsibility for key working participants during this stage. However, other members of the core multidisciplinary team and our associate practitioners contribute.

The nature of support is determined at the assessment stage, negotiated through the residential stage and is enacted against goal-orientated action plans during the subsequent 10–11 months. Needs vary between individuals and may range from telephone support during or following a flare up, to return to work management and support. Examples include our OTs undertaking work and home-based functional assessments, our physiotherapists supporting individuals in additional graded exercise programmes focused on functional goals, our nurses following up on sleep management, medication reductions and motivational and family work, and recently our psychologist offering guided work supported by telephone appointments with a patient who was struggling with thoughts and feelings following a return to the environment in which his accident happened. We also liaise with disability employment advisors, vocational consultants, occupational health nurses, human resource mangers and others. As well as delivering ongoing support, the consultant nurses coordinate and maintain appropriate levels of contact with the participant, their GP, the referrer and colleagues.

Upon conclusion of the ongoing support stage, a final report is complied for the participant comparing entry and outcome scores, progress against goals and recommendations. The report is made available to those in the participant's community who require it to continue supporting the individual. The participant is then discharged.

Developing a PMP, whether in the independent or NHS sector, involves more than the clinical service. People need to know you are there in order to refer to you. Experience in the NHS meant we all knew that it can be challenging to get through to the right people to 'sell' the PMP service for the benefit of patients and their families, but we were not sure how to do this in the independent sector. Few health care practitioners, after all, have experience in marketing. This and other challenges are addressed in the following section.

Challenges in implementing the service

This section discusses further some of our key challenges in implementing our service. These include identification of red flags, managing referrals, marketing and managing the delivery and corporate business.

Identifying red flags

No development is challenge free. In an article in the *British Pain Society (BPS) Newsletter* in Spring 2006, the challenges we faced were discussed (Burrows 2006) with the identification of red flags among the first. The challenge of developing protocols to manage red flags was introduced in the previous section. The reality was that in parallel to the PMP we were also developing two other levels of service – 'brief interventions' and 'pain education programmes'. We had begun admitting to these services and three of our first eight patients had red flags (New Zealand Guidelines Group and ACC 2003). One patient was suspected of having red flags during the initial self-referral telephone call when he described being diagnosed with thoracic osteoporosis 6 months previously. He was seen that day and following assessment the GP was contacted. The patient was referred to a haematologist the day after and sadly died from multiple myeloma 6 weeks later. Another, referred to us by a GP required orthopaedic surgery that was successfully undertaken within a week. The third was less clear-cut. However, by this time we had secured direct referral rights to a number of consultants in pain around the UK. The individual was seen quickly, the problem diagnosed and a combination of medical pain management and surgery resolved the issue.

ANP is not solely dependent upon clinical knowledge and expertise. Knowing the red flags list does not mean that as a nurse, you are capable of accurately and consistently recognising red flags in clinical practice. While experience and intuition (which is recognised as part of expert practice) can help (Benner & Tanner 1987; Manley *et al.* 2005), the ANP needs to have clear protocols for onward liaison and referral if safety is to be assured. One of the local consultants in pain raised this point and in an appropriately challenging conversation reassured himself that we had, through my leadership, given careful consideration to the necessary strategies. It was this debate that led to us being given direct referral rights, a position that is not only professionally reassuring, but also of significant importance for patient safety. Whilst these experiences can be uncomfortable and challenging, it enhanced the confidence of the team in considering opening up referral routes to the NHS PMP to which we contribute.

Managing referrals

One of the implications of the protocol is that to date all referrals have come through myself. As the organisation grows, the apparent reality is that we will have to find an alternative. A colleague consultant nurse is now confident to take referrals. However, the actuality is that as our referrals have grown the pattern has changed. The large majority of referrals now come via solicitors, case management and insurance companies, and potential participants have been screened for red flags.

The change in referral patterns has brought its own challenges. Our main market is not the early intervention that we had envisaged. Most of our participants are between 1 and 3 years into their pain journeys. They have typically been involved in accidents at work or on the road, have active or recently settled medico-legal cases, are often complex and require a different level of input than that originally planned. Approximately half are in work, though often struggling, while the remainder are on long-term sick leave or have been medically retired. As a consequence, we have and are continuing to develop our PMP. The clinical developments are addressed later in this chapter, the marketing challenges are considered here.

Marketing your service

According to the Chartered Institute of Marketing, marketing is 'the management process responsible for identifying, anticipating and satisfying customer requirements profitably.' This starts with everyone understanding and 'living' the mission statement, which is part of the business culture.

We offer three levels of clinical services:

- Brief interventions generally focused upon one or two therapeutic interventions for patients with acute or chronic pain.
- PEPs generally delivered by one or at the most two practitioners (nurse or therapist) in the client's home or place of work. Based upon the principles of CBT and drawing upon the materials and resources of the PMP, PEPs are suitable for people who do not require or cannot access the PMP.
- The third level is of course the PMP.

There is good evidence for the efficacy of CBT-based PMPs in improving pain experience, mood, coping, negative outlook on pain and activity levels (Morley *et al.* 1999;

van Tulder *et al.* 2000; Guzmán *et al.* 2001; Hoffman *et al.* 2007). The evidence base is part of marketing and is important when we explain our service. Over time we have trained ourselves not just to live our philosophies, but also to be able to articulate them quickly and succinctly when faced with enquiries. We work hard to ensure our materials, whether paper, web-based or verbal are consistent. Much of this activity is led conjointly by the marketing director and myself, as although the responsibility lies with the marketing director, the professional accountability remains with me.

Our biggest marketing challenge was to identify who our referrers might be and to access them. The clinical team had many excellent ideas, but little expertise. Informal contact for advice, with a friend with marketing experience, resulted in them becoming our marketing manager. Despite this we continued to struggle. The market we had perceived – given that 1:7 have persistent pain – was 'not there'. We were ahead of our time. We now have a clear strategy: networking, investing in our market through training and education, spending time 'account managing' and making best use of changes in rehabilitation guidance and other contextual developments.

A further challenge has been 'marketing' our assessment process. Potential participants enjoy the flexibility, welcoming us into their homes across the UK or appreciating that telephone assessments can be carried out anytime between 8 a.m. and 9 p.m., be halted if the individual needs a break and resume again 5–15 minutes later – thus enabling the person to pace. Referrers can initially be wary of telephone assessing. However, as we have become more skilled at both assessing in this way and in articulating the pros and cons, we are able to manage the queries competently and confidently.

Managing delivery

Delivery challenges are considered from a content perspective later as they tend to be driven by evaluation. Personal challenges are addressed here. Our residential programme can be personally exhausting – for the participants, practitioners and support staff. The evidence indicates that the more intense the programme, the better the outcomes appear to be. Individual appointments can start at 8 a.m. with group sessions commencing around 10 a.m. Evening sessions conclude anywhere from 7.15 p.m. to 8.15 p.m., practitioner discussions frequently follow. The support staff set up and break down the room on a weekly basis, deal with participant transport and non-clinical queries, provide additional resources as requested and man the office. The operations manager and her team coordinate the non-clinical endeavour and I focus on the clinical activity. Participants are frequently energised by the conclusion of the residential stage, but need careful support over the following fortnight to minimise the natural dip in motivation and enthusiasm that follows any group activity.

Our ongoing support offers a 'unique selling product', which on the one hand facilitates marketing, but on the other, sets up a lot of 'frequently asked questions' – precisely because it is out of the ordinary. Again, led by myself, we have had to train ourselves to articulate the clinical rationale for offering this service and the process that is followed. The community in this instance includes the participants and their families, the practitioners (core and associate teams), the support staff, referrers, GPs and, where relevant, employers. My role includes telephone and email liaison, with letters and formal reports the responsibility of the key worker, under my supervision.

Managing the business

Developing an independent nurse-led PMP in the community offers more than clinical challenges. As highlighted in the *BPS Newsletter* (Burrows 2006) there were business plans and policies to write, internal systems to develop, insurance policies to set up, data protection registration to organise and all the other factors required for running a business. In the early days, drawing upon personal experience, the advice of colleagues in the Royal College of Nursing's (RCN's) Nurse Entrepreneurs Group and in their publication 'Nurse entrepreneurs: turning initiative into independence', a new edition of which was published in 2007, was essential in the preparation. Additional advice was obtained from the bank manager, accountant and others referred to in Chapter 7. The structure of the company can be seen in Figure 9.1.

Developing an accounting system and costing our services was something of a challenge for a team who had predominantly worked within public service. Putting the actual figures together was not difficult, being confident that the fees were warranted because of service quality was more demanding. The physiotherapist was a great help having worked in independent practice for much of her career. We also received advice from a local PCT commissioner who was supportive of our developments.

It is interesting to note at this point the different qualities that other team members brought to the business – the psychologist has some excellent clinical development ideas, the OT is very good at identifying governance issues, the medical consultant has a keen eye for business regulation, one of the other consultant nurses is incredibly contextually aware, flagging up national and international developments we need to consider, a further consultant nurse is dedicated to ensuring that the accuracy and quality of materials is second to none. Everyone – practitioners and support team – is marvellously flexible. The challenge in leading the team is managing the enthusiasm and ideas in a business sensible and clinically progressive manner.

There is one person I have not mentioned a great deal but the business would not have survived without our operations manager. Setting up a new service is time-consuming and costly. Whether in the NHS or independent sector, finances are finite and have to be juggled. Our operations manager is a juggler par excellence. The skills we have learnt in the independent sector have made us more aware of cost-effectiveness with our NHS programmes, and I do mean here the ability to provide an effective service at an appropriate cost. ANPs are faced with exciting opportunities. Understanding business like financial management and the way in which it can support a quality service is paramount whatever the sector one is operating in.

Maintaining standards and evaluating the service

Many years ago the author had a particular interest in approaches to evaluating academic professional curricula (Burrows 1991). She has undertaken service evaluation

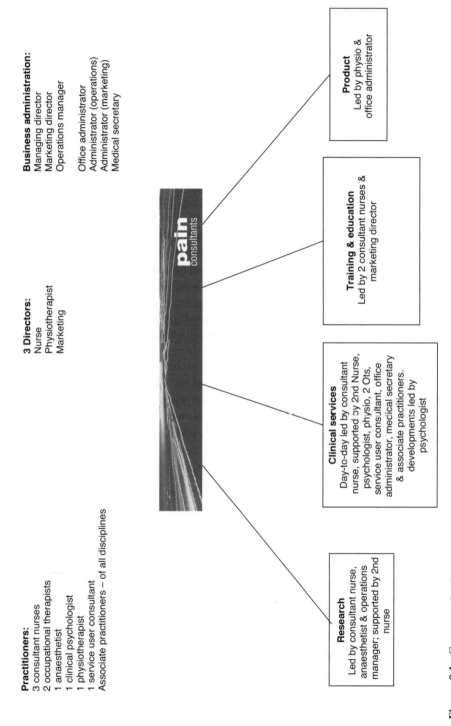

Business administration:
Managing director
Marketing director
Operations manager

Office administrator
Administrator (operations)
Administrator (marketing)
Medical secretary

3 Directors:
Nurse
Physiotherapist
Marketing

Practitioners:
3 consultant nurses
2 occupational therapists
1 anaesthetist
1 clinical psychologist
1 physiotherapist
1 service user consultant
Associate practitioners – of all disciplines

pain consultants

Product
Led by physio &
office administrator

Training & education
Led by 2 consultant nurses &
marketing director

Clinical services
Day-to-day led by consultant
nurse, supported by 2nd Nurse,
psychologist, physio, 2 Ots,
service user consultant, office
administrator, medical secretary
& associate practitioners.
developments led by
psychologist

Research
Led by consultant nurse,
anaesthetist & operations
manager; supported by 2nd
nurse

Figure 9.1 Company structure.

research and more recently an NHS PMP audit (Burrows *et al.* 2006). She values integrity and believes that quality is in the detail. In the BPS article, she highlighted that NHS practitioners have in the past questioned whether governance systems in the independent sector can be as good as the NHS (Burrows 2006). It is true that our systems and arrangements are considerably less complex than those in the NHS; however, they must be and are just as rigorous – after all our livelihoods depend on it on a day-to-day basis. This section outlines our approaches to maintaining standards and how we evaluate our services.

Governance is 'the set of arrangements or system by which the affairs of the organisation are ordered and monitored' (see Chapter 4). We have systems in place for corporate management, finance management, human resources, IT and staff development; we have strategies for marketing and service development; we have protocols for clinical delivery, research, product management and our training and education services; we have policies on access to health records, data protection, copyright clearance, confidentiality, lone working and staff sickness among others; we have codes for professional conduct and procedures for dealing with complaints, disciplinary and grievance matters; we have a multiplicity of insurances.

Some of the above have been written by myself, some by other members of the team and some, such as the disciplinary and grievance procedures are downloaded from public organisations. We have a list available and include copies of individual documents in appropriate locations. For example, the PMP manual includes clinically relevant policies. Our systems are thus open to scrutiny by our community – the team, participants, our referrers and clients, our accountants, bank manager, tax and VAT inspectors and so on. The responsibility for much of this lies with the operations manager, but the final accountability is with the directors.

The remainder of this section focuses upon some aspects of clinical, rather than corporate governance. However, before doing so, attention is drawn to the section on professional indemnity insurance in Chapter 7. In addition to individual indemnity through their Royal Colleges, our practitioners – and thus participants – are covered through insurance held by the organisation.

Clinical governance

Clinical governance includes the criteria outlined in Table 9.2.

In relation to patient, public and carer involvement, as previously mentioned, a service user consultant was involved in the PMP development. As with many PMPs we have past participants come and talk to the groups contributing to a graduate session and a session on managing pain in the work place. We encourage carers to be involved at the assessment stage and during ongoing support. Adult carers are also involved in our research programme, which focuses upon the impact of pain upon them.

As with other PMPs, our participants evaluate the group sessions verbally and in writing. We also ask them about their experiences and suggestions for the assessment and ongoing support stages. We collate testimonials and publish these appropriately.

Table 9.2   Clinical governance criteria

Patient, public and carer involvement	Analysis of patient's professional involvement and interaction, and strategy, planning and delivery of care
Strategic capacity and capability	Planning, communication and governance arrangements, and cultural behaviour aspects
Risk management	Incident reporting, infection control, prevention and control of risk
Staff management and performance	Recruitment, workforce planning, appraisals
Education, training and continuous professional development	Professional re-validation, management development, confidentiality and data protection
Clinical effectiveness	Clinical audit management, planning and monitoring, learning through research and audit
Information management	Patient records, etc.
Communication	Patient and public, external partners, internal, board and organisation wide
Leadership	Throughout the organisation, including board, chair and non-executive directors, chief executive and executive directors, managers and clinicians.
Team working	Within the service, senior managers, clinical and multidisciplinary teams, and across organisations

Source: Reproduced under the terms of the Click-Use licence.

I would say that we also collate complaints and investigate according to our policy; however, while the policy is in place, we have never had to enact it.

We have received some encouraging feedback from participants in all three levels of our clinical service, much of which has been made public as required by the communication aspect of clinical governance. One participant, who had been an international marketing manager, contacted a journalist and had her story and progress covered in a series of articles. This lady has also appeared in a company DVD and her picture is on the front of our clinical services leaflets. Other participants have spoken at our conferences – not about the service, but about themselves. Their willingness to engage in these activities is, we believe, a positive reflection on our service. However, it has also meant that we have had to develop confidentiality agreements and obtain signed permission to use people's personal information or appearances in DVDs and so on to meet data protection requirements as well as our own internal governance standards.

Our information management includes maintaining a practice list that is updated each time we receive a new referral or discharge a participant. The list not only contains the individual's name, date of birth, clinic number, referrer details and so on, but also their main pain problem, treatment focus and summary of outcome. It thus forms a useful basis for our main annual audit. We have a 'practice list action points' document updated on a weekly basis by the consultant nurses to support key worker activity. This is a relatively new development, reflecting growth and the need to ensure all our participants treatment and communication needs are being managed in a timely fashion. Our clinical services administrator also receives a copy so that she is able to respond to enquiries from participants and referrers. Participants, of course, also have clinical notes files.

We prepare a considerable number of lengthy reports – at assessment, following the residential stage and three monthly thereafter to the point of discharge. In addition, there are letters to GPs and other practitioners involved in the participant's health, social and work management. We use emails and texts. The latter are transcribed and filed in the participant's notes. Again it is the consultant nurses' responsibility – in collaboration with the clinical services administrator and our medical secretary – to ensure that participant records are up-to-date and transparent should the participant or other authorities wish to view them. Because many of our participants have active medico-legal cases, we can be asked to forward copies of the clinical notes, with participants' permission, to solicitors. Our record keeping is fulsome and carried out according to NHS standards.

Corporate and clinical audit

Clinical audit is an ongoing process and the responsibility lies with myself and delegated assistance. Clinical and corporate reports are produced for every board meeting. A full clinical audit is undertaken at the end of each financial year. The audit report focuses upon treatment outcomes. Because our service is relatively new (and participant numbers thus relatively small) we are moving towards, rather than actually being able to currently provide comparisons of outcomes. This position should alter by the time the next annual audit is due in March 2009. The report also provides an update on general clinical activity, staff training and academic consultancy.

Staff training is an area we invest in. Most recently the team, together with one of our OT associates, came together for an internal training day facilitated by our Clinical Psychologist. The focus was on a new area of therapeutic practice and one that the team hopes to move forward in developing over the coming year. All core and associate staff are offered gratis places at our conferences, and we also fund staff development activities at external meetings and study days. Responsibility for determining attendance is held by myself in terms of clinical rationale and by the operations manager for the financial support.

Our corporate systems are reviewed by an external business consultant in December each year. This provides useful critique from a fresh pair of eyes, as well as mentorship for the directors and operations manager. Corporate goals are determined for the coming 12 months. The operations manager works closely with the directors and accountants to ensure progress against business aims is evaluated on a quarterly basis. This process is not just good business practice; it is also about teamwork. Benson and Rice (2007) highlight that for leadership to be perceived as rewarding, gaining support is paramount. Their work on the NHS Clinical Teams Programme (CTP) suggested four sources: those in a similar position, i.e. other leaders and innovators, team colleagues, local managers and the CTP facilitators. In various ways, I (and business) obtain support in each of the first three categories albeit in a different context.

We have a relatively flat hierarchy, thus practitioners and business staff are expected to lead on some aspects and work as team members in others.

Justifying the advanced nursing contribution

Throughout this chapter, I have attempted to highlight the contribution to the development of a nurse-led PMP. As an ANP, I have led and motivated the team, used my clinical expertise, enhanced my corporate skills, developed business skills and employed a marketing manager. Knowing yourself and being able to analyse your organisations is the first of Wallace's (2004) skill acquisition areas and a key component of any successful development activity (see Chapter 7). Knowing that the practitioner team did not possess sufficient marketing, knowledge and skills were key to making that decision.

The RCN (2008) describes a number of core elements to the ANP role. The first of these is the ability to make professionally autonomous decisions for which he or she is accountable. In the development outlined in this chapter, the practitioner and business staff work as a team. Each member is also responsible for decision-making in their area – but perhaps not always autonomously. In a PMP there is a lot of joint formulation, delivery and decision-making. However, practitioners make autonomous decisions, using their clinical expertise. Autonomy involves dealing with the unexpected. Recently I made a decision to 'suspend' ongoing support for one of our participants as he has a number of other health issues that have greater priority. By suspending support, we will be able to work with him again at a more appropriate time. The need to suspend was a clinically autonomous decision. Actually doing so was my responsibility as managing director as there will be unfunded costs to the company. ANPs need the confidence to balance clinical decision-making in the context of wider implications.

By taking referrals and holding responsibility in assessment on behalf of the team, I 'receive patients with undifferentiated and undiagnosed problems' and exercises skills such as physical examination (RCN 1983). Many clinical nurse specialists in pain management fulfil this criterion for ANP practice on a daily basis. The third criterion involves screening for risk factors – a process outlined by this ANP in relation to the identification of red flags. Fourthly, I make differential diagnoses in relation to pain and its impact using decision-making and problem-solving skills. Developing ongoing pain management plans in liaison with participants, I provide treatment as an individual and as part of the team. I also refer to other agencies, support participants in managing their pain, provide health education in relation to the impact of pain and have the authority to admit and discharge patients. Working collaboratively within and outside of the team, I provide consultancy internally and externally to the organisation, as well as being the team leader.

Opportunities for developing as an ANP in pain management are increasing both in the NHS and in the independent sector. Primary care, social care and vocational rehabilitation developments enable those with ideas to explore and implement new initiatives. In doing so, ANPs need to be 'politically' and clinically aware of national developments. In working on one's own developments, ANPs need to know themselves and their organisation, plan their strategy, understand constraints and be aware of resources (Wallace 2004). The most important resource is within ourselves – our knowledge, skills and capacity for action.

Conclusions

This chapter has shown how an ANP can take on a leadership role in developing a PMP in the community. Many of the concepts discussed are of course equally appropriate to other service development by nurses across the pain arena. Many ANPs will already possess the necessary knowledge and skills. By considering the range of opportunities that exist from new and differing perspectives, ANPs have the potential to enhance services for the benefit of people with pain, their families and the community at large.

Appendix 1

Red flags indicative of possible serious spinal pathology

- Age under 20, over 55
- Non-mechanical pain
- Thoracic pain
- History of cancer, steroids, HIV
- Unwell, weight loss
- Widespread neurological signs and symptoms (S&S)
- Structural deformity
- Cauda equina (sphincter/gait disturbance, saddle anaesthesia)

Psychosocial yellow flags – the beliefs and behaviours which may predict poor outcome and which pain management programmes address

- Pain, harm/potential severe disablement
- Fear avoidance & reduced activity
- Low mood & social withdrawal
- Anticipates passive treatment, rather than active participation

(New Zealand Guidelines Group and ACC 2003).

Acknowledgements

My thanks to all in the PainConsultants team – practitioners (core and associate), business and support staff – without your hard work and commitment this venture would forever have remained a pipe dream. To our referrers, thank you for having confidence in us. To the people with pain, their families, GPs and employers with whom we work – you are our raison d'être.

References

Beck, A.T., Steer, R.A., Brown, G.K., 1996. *BDI-II, Beck Depression Inventory Manual*, 2nd edn. San Antonio: The Psychological Corporation, Harcourt Brace & Company.

Benner, P.C.A., Tanner, C., 1987. How expert nurses use intuition. *American Journal of Nursing*, 87(1), 23–31.

Benson, A., Rice, M. (eds), 2007. *Developing and Sustaining Effective Teams*. London: Royal College of Nursing.

Borrill, C., West, M., 2002. *Team Working and Effectiveness in Health Care: Findings from the Health Care Team Effectiveness Project*. Birmingham: Aston Centre for Health Service Organisation Research.

British Pain Society, 2007. Recommended guidelines for pain management programmes for adults. Available at http://www.britishpainsociety.org/pub_professional.htm#pmp [accessed 3 March 2009].

Burrows, D., 1991. *The Ways in Which a Nurse Teacher Can Evaluate His Or Her Teaching*. Internal Report. High Wycombe: Buckinghamshire College of Nursing & Midwifery.

Burrows, D. 2006. The art and science of independent practice – what is this nurse up to? *The British Pain Society Newsletter*, Spring, 26–27. Available at http://www.britishpainsociety. org/bps_nl_spring 2006.pdf [accessed 3 March 2009].

Burrows, D., Mackay, C., Cotter, I., 2006. *Amersham Pain Management Programme Data Audit*. Buckinghamshire Hospitals NHS Trust & Wycombe PCT . Unpublished.

Burrows, D., Wood, G., Cotter, I., 2005. *Medication Review Questionnaire for Pain Management Programmes, Version 1*. PainConsultants Limited. Available at www.admin@ painconsultants.co.uk.

Chronic Pain Policy Coalition, 2007. *A new pain manifesto*. Available at www. paincoalition.org.uk [accessed 3 March 2009].

Deacon, L., 2005. *Physical Activity Profile for Pain Management Programmes, Version 1*. PainConsultants Limited. Available at www.admin@painconsultants.co.uk.

Fordyce, W.E., Fowler, R., Lehmann, J., De Lateur, B., Sand, P., Trieschmann, R., 1973. Operant conditioning in the treatment of chronic pain. *Archives of Physical Medicine and Rehabilitation*, 54, 399–408.

Gilson, B.S., Gilson, J.S., Bergner, M., Bobbitt, R.A., Kressel, S., Pollard, W.E., Vesselago, M., 1975. The sickness impact profile: development of an outcome measure of health care. *AJPH*, 65(12), 1304–1310.

Green, L., 2006. Physiotherapy for musculoskeletal disorders. Available at http:// www.eastsussex.gov.uk/NR/rdonlyres/49268D27-350B-4B37-A1C5-3732209001E2/9841/ APPENDIX4PhysioBusinessCaseReporttoHRMB.pdf [accessed 3 March 2009].

Guzmán, J., Esmail, R., Karjalainen, K., Irvin, E., Bombardier, C., 2001. Multidisciplinary rehabilitation for chronic low back pain: systematic review. *British Medical Journal*, 322, 511–516.

Hoffman, B.M., Papas, R.K., Chatkoff, D.K., Kerns, R.D., 2007. Meta-analysis of psychological interventions for chronic low back pain. *Health Psychology*, 26, 1–9.

Main, C.J., Spanswick, C.C., 2000. *Pain Management: An Interdisciplinary Approach*. Edinburgh: Elsevier Health Sciences.

Manley, K., Hardy, S., Titchen, A., Garbett, R., McCormack, B., 2005. *Changing Patients' Worlds through Nursing Practice Expertise: Exploring Nursing Practice Expertise through Emancipatory Action Research and Fourth Generation Evaluation*. London: Royal College of Nursing.

Melzack, R., 1987. The short-form McGill Pain questionnaire. *Pain*, 30, 191–197.

Morley, S., Eccleston, C., Williams, A., 1999. Systematic review and meta-analysis of randomized controlled trials of cognitive behaviour therapy and behaviour therapy for chronic pain in adults, excluding headache. *Pain*, 80, 1–13.

New Zealand Guidelines Group and ACC, 2003. New Zealand acute back pain guide. Available at www.nzgg.org.nz/guidelines/0072/albp_guide_col.pdf [accessed 3 March 2009].

RCN, 2007. Nurse entrepreneurs: turning initiative into independence. Available at www.rcn.org.uk/__data/assets/pdf_file/0018/115632/003215.pdf [accessed 3 March 2009].

RCN, 2008. Advanced Nurse Practitioners – an RCN guide to the advanced nurse practitioner role, competencies and programme accreditation. Available at http://www.rcn.org.uk/__data/assets/pdf_file/0003/146478/003207.pdf [accessed 3 March 2009].

Rosential, A., Keefe, F., 1983. The use of coping strategies in chronic low back pain patients: relationship to patient characteristics and current adjustment. *Pain*, 17, 33–44.

Turk, D.C., Meichenbaum, D., Genest, M., 1983. *Pain and Behavioural Medicine: A Cognitive-behavioral Perspective*. New York: Guildford Press.

VA National Pain Outcomes Workgroup, 2003. *VHA Pain Outcomes Toolkit*. Washington: Department of Veterans Affairs.

Van Tulder, M.W., Ostelo, R., Vlaeyen, J.W.S., Linton, S.J., Morley, S.J., Assendelft, W.J., 2000. Behavioural treatment of chronic low back pain: a systematic review within the framework of the Cochrane Back Review Group. *Spine*, 25, 2688–2699.

Vowles, K.E., McCraken, L.M., 2008. Acceptance and values-based action in chronic pain: a study of treatment effectiveness and process. *Journal of Consulting and Clinical Psychology*, 76, 397–407.

Wallace, R., 2004. *Strategic Partnerships: An Entrepreneur's Guide to Joint Ventures and Alliances*. Chicago: Dearborn Trade.

Wicksell, R.K., Melin, L., Lekander, M., Olsson, G.L., 2009. Evaluating the effectiveness of exposure and acceptance strategies to improve functioning and quality of life in longstanding pediatric pain – a randomized controlled trial. *Pain*, 141, 248–257.

Zigmond, A.S., Snaith, R.P., 1983. The hospital anxiety and depression scale. *Acta Psychiatrica Scandinavica*, 67(6), 361–440.

Chapter 10
Nurse prescribing in acute and chronic pain management

Trudy Towell and Martin Christensen

Introduction

In the UK improving the patients' experience has been emphasised by Lord Darzi (2007) in his report, to the Department of Health (DH), which encouraged organisations and services to develop safe, fair and equitable care around the needs and choice of patients. Traditional clinical roles have already been challenged and broken down to allow nurses to work more flexibly with expanded skills, particularly in the area of prescribing (National Prescribing Centre 2001; DH 2006a). All nurse prescribers within a specialist pain service or within generic nursing roles need appropriate education, ongoing support and continuing professional development (CPD) material. It is helpful to have a brief historical review of the policy documents which led to these changes.

In 1979 the first case for nurse prescribing was presented to the Royal College of Nursing (RCN) by a group of district nurses wishing to enhance the care they were providing for patients (Jones 2004). From this came a stepwise movement towards the announcement in early May 2006 that independent nurse prescribers could prescribe from the whole British National Formulary (BNF). These nurses would be able to assess, diagnose and prescribe without reference to a medical practitioner. However, this journey has been long and arduous. In 1986, after lobbying from the RCN, the Cumberlege Report was commissioned by the then Department of Health and Social Security (DHSS), which reviewed community nursing and made recommendations that nurses be able to prescribe a limited formulary (DHSS 1986). This was followed by the first Crown Report (*Report of the Advisory Group on Nurse Prescribing*, DH 1989), which suggested that specific items may be prescribed, the groups of patients that would most benefit and also emphasised the improvement that nurse prescribing would make to patient care, for example saving time, improving communication and clarifying professional responsibilities between nurses and general practitioners (GPs) (Courtenay & Griffiths 2006). The Cumberlege (DHSS 1986) and Crown (DH 1989) reports led to the bringing of a private member's bill culminating in the Medicinal Products: Prescription by Nurses Act 1992, granting the ability to prescribe to specifically trained district nurses and health visitors. The problem here was that these prescriptions would be limited to wound dressings, non-drug items or those on the general sales list. With an amendment to this piece of legislation in 1994, saw the publication of the first Nurse Prescribers' Formulary and the setting up eight pilot sites for nurse prescribing (at the behest of the Treasury, concerned with cost) which was to later extend to all National Health Service (NHS) regions in England (McHale 2003; Jordan & Griffiths 2004; Warner 2005). However, the Advisory Group Report (DH 1989) was also the catalyst in the quest for alternative means of drug administration by nurses, for example the use of group protocols. Group protocols in this instance were seen as local agreements between doctors and nurses (usually in the primary care setting) whereby the nurse could give patients specific drugs without a prescription. However, this ran into difficulties when it emerged that it was an illegal interpretation of the Medicine Act 1968. As a result the government requested an investigation into the illegality of group protocols; the second Crown Report (DH 1999) heralded patient group directions (PGDs) and the guidelines for their implementation were set out in a NHS Executive Health Service Circular (DH, 2000a, 2000b; McHale 2003; Jones 2004). PGDs are described as written instructions for the administration of medicines to patients who are not previously known to a non-prescribing practitioner (DH 2000a).

The final part of the Crown Report (1999) was undertaken to review prescribing, supplying and administration of medicines and as a result proposed a new framework. This new framework identified new categories of prescribers – independent and dependant (subsequently supplementary prescribers) – and new groups of health professional that could become prescribers (DH 1999). Up until this point these changes in prescribing legislation plus the governments agenda to alleviate emergency department waiting times and provide more community-based care led to the development of 'nurse-led' walk-in centres and minor injury units which required nurses to be able to assess, diagnose and prescribe. In 2001 the extended nurse prescribers' formulary was announced with its focus for nurses working in the areas of minor illness and injury, health promotion and palliative care (pain control). The new categories of independent and supplementary prescribers was endorsed in 2001 with supplementary prescribing coming into being in 2003 (Baird 2005), yet it would be another 3 years before nurses would be able to prescribe independently. Supplementary prescribers (nurses and pharmacists) must prescribe in conjunction with an independent prescriber, can prescribe any medication with the exception of controlled drugs as long as it is within the terms of a patient-specific clinical management plan following a diagnosis by the independent prescriber and must have completed relevant training (DH 2003). Finally in early May 2006 the Nurses Extended Formulary was discontinued and became the nurse independent prescribers enabling nurses to prescribe from the whole BNF for any clinical condition within their area of competence including some controlled drugs (DH 2006b).

Nurse prescribing commenced after the 1986 Cumberlege Report recommended that community nurses should be able to prescribe a limited list of items, followed by the Crown Report 1989 which led to the Nurse Prescribers Formulary for suitably qualified nurses to prescribe from. After pilot studies there was a national roll-out of nurse prescribing in 1998. The training required at this time to become an independent nurse prescriber included a distance learning package, a 3-day training course and assessment by written examination. The second Crown Report (1999) extended prescribing rights to include other groups such as nurses and pharmacists. The NHS Plan (2000) supported extending the prescribing authority, empowering front line staff detailed within shifting the balance of power.

It was envisaged that by 2004 the majority of nurses should be able to prescribe medicines independently, or as supplementary prescribers, or supply, or administer medicines under PGDs. PGDs first came to light after the first Nurse Prescriber's Formulary; however, it was the second Crown Report (DH 1999) that heralded the introduction of PGDs. Final amendments to the report not only identified new categories of prescribers, but together with the NHS Executive Health Service Circular (DH 2000a) were guidelines for PGD use and implementation acknowledged. This meant that there now existed a legal framework for which nurses could prescribe albeit limitedly. By definition, PGDs are written instructions that allow for the supply, sale and administration of named medicines to individuals that are unidentified at the time of treatment for a specific clinical situation without the need for a prescription (Baird & Morgan 2000; National Prescribing Centre (NPC) 2003).

Acute pain

University courses for independent and supplementary nurse prescribing were developed throughout the country in response to the NHS Plan (2000). These opened opportunities for improving acute pain management through initiatives such as:

- PGDs allowing ward nurses/emergency nurses to administer simple analgesia such as paracetamol (see National prescribing website www.npc.co.uk).
- PGDs for Entonox resulted in an increase in its use to support patients through difficult wound dressing changes, removal of drains or other short-term incident pains.
- Acute pain specialist nurses used PGDs to administer epidural boluses of bupivacaine for patients with severe breakthrough pain (but opiates are not allowed to be administered via a PGD).
- Acute pain specialist nurse prescribers were able to choose from an extended list (see Table 10.1).

Chronic pain

Independent prescribing for palliative care patients allowed nurse prescribers to choose from an extended list (see Table 10.2).

Specialist nurses working with patients experiencing chronic benign pain are prescribing medications such as demonstrated in Table 10.3.

Chronic benign pain is not recognised as palliative care, so opiates can only be prescribed by supplementary prescribing using a clinical management plan for these patients.

The complex and dynamic national non-medical prescribing standards and guidelines require a local overall strategy for improving the management of medicines and the development of nurse prescribing within pain services for patients in acute or chronic pain. Prescribing is not just writing a prescription. Considerations include the latest national developments, legal implications, medication risks versus the benefits

Table 10.1   Prescribing only medications in the nurse prescribers extended formulary, useful for acute pain

Analgesics
  Aspirin (*po*)
  Codeine phosphate (*po*)
  Diclofenac potassium (*po*)
  Diclofenac (*po/pr*/ophthalmic)
  Dihydrocodeine tartrate (*po*)
  Felbinac (external)
  Flurbiprofen (lozenges)
  Ibuprofen (external/*po*)
  Ibuprofen lysine (*po*)
  Ketoprofen (external)
  Nefopam (*po*)
  Paracetamol (*po*)
  Piroxicam (external)

Antiemetics
  Cyclizine (*po*/parenteral)
  Dolasetron (*po*/parenteral)
  Domperidone (*po/pr*)
  Granisetron (parenteral)
  Metoclopramide (*po*/parenteral)
  Ondansetron (*po*/parenteral)

of the prescription, the latest evidence base and consideration of the patient's information and education required to ensure compliance. An example of one large university teaching hospitals' strategy will be shared. This service and practice development is multifaceted and includes the rationale for development, the organisational policies, corporate steering groups, local medicine guidelines, national guidelines, implementation support with group multidisciplinary clinical supervision and CPD.

Table 10.2   Prescribing only medications in the nurse prescribers extended formulary, useful for chronic pain

Amitriptyline – palliative care
Baclofen (*po*) – palliative care
Dantolene (*po*) – palliative care
Gabapentin (*po*) – palliative care
Imipramine – palliative care
Nortriptyline – palliative care
Controlled drugs
  Morphine sulphate (*po*/parenteral/*pr*)[a]
  Morphine hydrochloride (*pr*)
  Diamorphine (*po*/parenteral)[a]
  Buprenorphine (transdermal) – palliative care
  Fentanyl (transdermal) – palliative care
  Oxycodone (*po*/parenteral) – palliative care

[a]For pain relief in respect of suspected myocardial infarction, or for relief of acute or severe pain after trauma including in either case post-operative pain relief.

Table 10.3 Examples of medication for specialist nurses using supplementary prescribing for patients experiencing chronic benign pain

Group	Drugs	Dose schedule	Comments	Reasons for referral back to independent prescriber
Antidepressant	Amitriptyline	10–150 mg nocte	Outside license	cardiovascular side effects, e.g. ECG changes, arrhythmias, postural hypotension, tachycardia
Anticonvulsant	Gabapentin	300–600 mg tds		headache, urinary incontinence, deranged liver function tests (LFTs)

Rationale for service development

Improving the patients' pain relief in hospital

Inadequate post-operative pain management has been reported for over 30 years in the UK (Marks & Sachar 1973; Fagerhaugh & Strauss 1977; Svensson *et al.* 2000), with similar findings in Hong Kong (Chung & Lui 2003), Australia and Canada (VanDenKerkhof & Goldstein 2004) to name only a few. Specialist nurses working in hospital environments understand the complexity of the barriers to patients obtaining excellent pain relief.

During daily visits to the wards, specialist nurses provide education to ward nurses, junior doctors, patients and their relatives, during their consultations and assessments of patients in pain. Frequently, there is a lack of systematic pain assessment, a lack of analgesics prescribed by junior doctors, a lack of equipment such as patient-controlled analgesia devices (Picker Institute Europe Reports 2002, 2004) and a lack of planning for epidural or intravenous patient-controlled, step-down analgesia. Often patients have to wait up to 24 hours for the junior doctors to prescribe the analgesics recommended by the specialist nurses.

Local audit (Bennett 2005) demonstrated a large variation between the younger adult (2–3 hours wait) and the elderly patients (6–8 hours wait) in obtaining analgesia after admission to hospital in medical environments. Gregory and Bramwell (2008) pilot project allowing Oramorph to be administered with one nurse's signature in the CD register led to patients waiting less time to receive their analgesia. No nurse wanted to return to the traditional two-nurse checking of Oramorph. Specialist nurses in acute pain services are provided with the opportunity to train and support ward-based nurses with projects for improving the timely administration of analgesics. They can also develop themselves by attending a university course in non-medical prescribing to support the provision of timely, appropriate prescriptions to provide a higher standard of care to patients. Even though the World Health Organization's (WHO's) three-step ladder has improved the treatment of pain throughout the world, we still find studies reporting ineffective analgesia (Bach 2007). Nurse prescribing provides an opportunity to improve this and subsequently the patients' experience.

Improving the patients' pain relief in the community

In the hospital outpatient chronic pain clinics, patients often describe difficulties in getting an appointment with their GP, sometimes waiting for up to 2 weeks. This leads to patient delays in obtaining analgesics and continued pain and suffering. Others describe non-compliance with the consultant advised trials of medications. All patients recommended for strong opiate medication, require comprehensive biopsychosocial assessment, education, monitoring and evaluation as advised by the British Pain Society guidelines (BPS 2004).

Tomorrow's primary care trusts need specialist nurses to help provide multipurpose clinics or polyclinics to move hospital-based chronic pain services and enhance primary care provision (Bence 2008). The government policies including nurse prescribing support the change in services to deliver care closer to the patients' home. Long-term conditions management such as patients with chronic pain will be managed by teams of GPs, but they lack specialist pain knowledge, providing opportunities for specialist nurses to work with them and develop pain clinics in the community settings.

Organisational agreement for service development

A framework for non-medical prescribing rights was further developed and approved by Nottingham University Hospital Medicines Management Committee and subgroup Non-Medical Prescribing, Administration and Supply Group (NUH-NMPAS 2007). This operational policy is related to both independent and supplementary prescribing and included a clinical management plan template (see Figure 10.1), a specimen signature form for the pharmacy department records and a directorate independent nurse prescribing agreement which included the names of consultants, the list of licensed medicines (formulated by the non-medical prescriber) together with doses/indications specified in ratified local guidelines, national guidelines or current BNF. Off-label prescribing of licensed medicines is also permitted if referred to in local guidelines, national guidelines or current BNF (DH 2005, 2006).

The policy states that all prescribing practices must adhere to the legal requirements and national guidance. The framework ensures that risks of error are minimised by adhering to the local health community overarching framework. The non-medical prescribing, administration and supply of medicines group meets on a monthly basis. The group has evolved over a 2-year period, when the two hospital trusts merged into one. Differences in two hospital policies were overcome by multiprofessionals agreeing to join the NMPAS group and work together to merge and develop one trust policy.

The group consists of:

- Chair – nurse lead (2006–2008 Trudy Towell);
- Two medical members from each of the trusts' two campuses (included two consultant anaesthetists, a consultant renal physician and a consultant for the elderly);

Addressograph label **or** Name: Date of Birth: Hospital number:	Drug allergy or If none known tick box adverse effect: ☐
Independent prescriber(s):	Supplementary prescriber(s):
Condition(s) to be treated	Aim of treatment

Guidelines or protocols supporting this Clinical Management Plan

Medicines selected from the guideline or protocol and prescribed by the SP:

Preparation	Indication	Dose schedule	Reasons for referral back to the IP

If no guideline or protocol supporting this CMP, medicines that may be prescribed by the SP

Preparation	Indication	Dose schedule	Specific indications for referral back to IP

Frequency of review and monitoring by:

Supplementary prescriber	Independent prescriber +/– supplementary prescriber

ADR reported to CSM / copy sent to Medicines Information State drug(s) and reaction involved

Date for review of CMP: (must be at least at 12 months)

Agreed by independent prescribers(s) Sign and print name(s)	Date	Agreed by supplementary prescriber(s) Sign and print name(s)	Date	Date agreed with patient/carer

Figure 10.1 Supplementary prescribing clinical management plan template (see www.npc.org). (Reproduced with kind permission of © NUH NHS Trust.)

- Two senior pharmacists (one senior pharmacist with special responsibility for PGDs/databases);
- One non-medical prescriber or practice development nurse from each of the trusts (nine) directorates.

This group coordinates and supports the processes required for the development, ratification and implementation of PGDs (see Figure 10.2) and non-medical independent and supplementary prescribing. The group supports safe practice by identifying

1. Clinical situation to which this patient group direction applies

i	*Definition of the clinical condition/situation*
ii	*Inclusion criteria*
iii	*Exclusion criteria*
iv	*Actions for patients excluded from treatment*
v	*Actions for patients not wishing to receive care*

2. Characteristics of staff authorised to administer/supply medicines under this patient group direction

i	*Professional qualifications required* Registered nurse(RN)The registered nurse must possess valid registration with the Nursing and Midwifery Council (NMC)
ii & iii	*Specialist qualifications, training and experience relevant to the clinical condition and the medicines used* Any nurse *administering/supplying* ....under this direction must in addition to 2(i) above
iv	*Requirements for continued training* All nurses acting under this direction will be expected to maintain knowledge and competence as defined by the NMC's (2004) Standards for Post –Registration Education and Practice

3. Description of medicines available in the Patient Group Direction

(i) Drug to be supplied	(iii) Legal status	(iv) Dose to be given	(v) Route	(vi) Frequency	(vii) Total dose/ number of treatments

(ii) Drug to be administered	(iii) Legal status	(iv) Dose to be given	(v) Houte	(vi) Frequency	(vii) Total dose/ number of treatments

viii	*Information about follow-up treatment*
ix	*Advice to the patient before or after treatment*
x	*Instructions for identifying and managing future possible adverse outcomes*
xi	*Referral for medical advice*
xii	*Facilities and supplies that should be available*
xiii	*Treatment records*
xiv	*Special considerations relating to the administration of concurrent medicines*

Figure 10.2 Patient group direction template for Nottingham University Hospitals (see www.npc.org). (Reproduced with kind permission of © NUH NHS Trust.)

	4. Management and monitoring of Patient Group Directions
i	*Names of the professionals drawing up this Patient Group Direction* *Person, or their successor, responsible for ensuring that only fully competent, qualified and trained professionals operate within directions.
ii	*Signature of professional named as responsible and clinical director* Name: Named Professional Signed: Date: Name: Clinical Director Signed: Date:
iii	*For office use only* *Signature of authorising pharmacist* Name Signed: Date *Signature of authorising committee;* *Chair of NMPAS or MMC* Name: Signed: Date;
iv	*Expected review date (2 years from ratification):*

Directorate
Title of the Direction

Printed names	Date	Signature

Figure 10.2   (*Continued*)

and addressing risk factors along with mechanisms for auditing outcomes. Issues which require the advice or authorisation from the medicines management committee are referred on to that group. All non-medical prescribers were invited to attend the meeting when their PGDs or independent/supplementary prescribing agreements were submitted for ratification. The nurses found the supportive group, encouraging, challenging and valued the educational experience.

Selecting nursing roles suitable for non-medical prescribing must demonstrate improvements in patient benefits such as more efficient access to medicines. Nominations are then forwarded to the local universities offering the independent and supplementary prescribing education programme. The trust matrons ensure that nominated nurses have the ability to study at degree level and can undertake self-directed learning. Each nurse has at least 3 years' post-registration experience and 1 year in the clinical area of which they intend to practice. An identified doctor agrees to contribute to and supervise the 12 days' learning in practice. The nursing post must have the opportunity for independent or supplementary prescribing and the matron ensures the nurse can have access to CPD opportunities after finishing the course and agrees to inclusion of the role within the individual's job description.

The hospital's Medicines Code of Practice outlines the responsibilities for practitioners – nurses, pharmacists and doctors – to only prescribe in their area of competence, and for non-medical prescribers, only those drugs named on their independent prescribing agreement (see Table 10.4). The supplementary prescribers may only prescribe if there is a valid clinical management plan.

The policy for non-medical prescribing describes the responsibilities of the independent, the supplementary, the independent medical prescriber and the requirements for clinical management plans.

Prescriptions

The specialist nurses in acute or chronic pain use four methods to prescribe:

- Inpatients – drug prescription and administration record.
- Outpatients' prescription form where the hospital pharmacy dispenses the prescription; only used if the patients' visit to their GP is delayed.
- Outpatients' FP10HP prescription where the community pharmacist dispenses the prescription; only used if the patients' visit to their GP is delayed.
- Yellow form providing prescribing advice to the GP.

The FP10HP prescriptions require the prescriber to use a stamp which states 'NMC independent/supplementary prescriber NMC No. and hospital address, contact number and Prescription Pricing Authority (PPA) approved prescribing account code in the address box'. The prescriptions are pre-stamped by pharmacy at the top of the prescribing area. All consultations and prescription information is then recorded in the medical and nursing notes. The rationale for this is recommended as good practice by the DH (DH 2005, 2006).

Evaluation use of audit and CPD

Each nurse audits their own practice and provides an annual report to their matron or chief pharmacist. All nurses forward a copy to the hospital nursing department/trust lead for non-medical prescribing. Requirements of their audit include the safety evaluation, effectiveness, appropriateness and patient's acceptability.

It is recommended that each prescriber plans for CPD, which reflects and includes:

- National Prescribing Centre guidance (NPC 2001);
- Clinical supervision sessions, individually or in groups;

Table 10.4 Examples extracted from the clinical guidelines for non-medical prescribing in the Pain Management Service Nottingham University Hospitals NHS Trust

Drug group	BNF class	Drug	Rx type	Legal classification	Administration route	Dose schedule	Notes	Specific indication for referral to independent prescriber
Laxatives	1.6.2	Senna	IP/SP	P	Oral	15–30 mg sennosides daily (i.e. 2–4 tablets or 10–20 mL syrup)		Suspected intestinal obstruction; atonic non-functioning colon; hypokalaemia
Antidepressants	4.3.1	Amitriptyline	SP	POM	Oral	10–150 mg daily	Outside PL Neuropathic pain Sleep hygiene First-line TCA	Ischaemic heart disease; cardiovascular side effects (e.g. ECG changes, arrhythmias); convulsions; hyponatraemia
Drugs used in nausea and vomiting	4.6	Cyclizine	IP/SP	POM	Oral/IV	50 mg tds	See local guideline	Urinary retention; prostatic hypertrophy; extra pyramidal adverse effects
		Prochlorperazine	IP/SP	POM	Buccal	3–6 mg bd	Buccal route. See local guideline	Extra pyramidal adverse effects; respiratory depression
		Ondansetron	IP/SP	POM	IV	4 mg stat dose	Pruritis. See local guideline	

(*Continued*)

Table 10.4 (*Continued*)

Drug group	BNF class	Drug	Rx type	Legal classification	Administration route	Dose schedule	Notes	Specific indication for referral to independent prescriber
Non-opioid analgesics	4.7.1	Paracetamol	IP/SP	GSL/P/POM	Oral/IV	1 g qds	Oral route IV only if oral route unavailable	Rash; blood disorders
		Nefopam	IP/SP	POM	Oral	30–90 mg tds		Nausea; urinary retention; light headedness
Opioid analgesics	4.7.2	Morphine (IV) bolus	IP	CD POM	IV	10 mg loading dose in 2 mg increments every 5 minutes with appropriate monitoring available (acute post-operative pain/trauma)	See local protocol (intravenous algorithm)	
		Morphine (IV) PCA	IP	CD POM	IV	1– 2 mg bolus 5 minutes lockout +/– background infusion up to 2 mg/hour where appropriate monitoring available (acute post-operative pain/trauma)	In conjunction with local protocol (IV PCA)	
		Morphine (SC)	IP	CD POM	SC	10 mg hourly	See local protocol (subcutaneous algorithm)	

		Drug	Prescriber	Legal status	Route	Dose	Notes	Side effects
		Tramadol (Oral)	IP/SP	POM	Oral	50–100 mg qds	Maximum 600 mg daily Licensed maximum daily dose 400 mg	Convulsions; excessive sedation; dependence; marked hypotension
		Dihydrocodeine	IP/SP	POM	Oral	30–60 mg qds	Maximum 240 mg daily	Excessive sedation; dependence
Antiepileptics		Gabapentin	IP/SP	POM	Oral	300–600 mg tds	Dose titration required Maximim dose 2400 mg daily Maximum licensed dose for neuropathic pain 1800 mg daily	Hallucinations and pyschosis; pancreatitis, urinary incontinence
		Pregabalin	IP/SP	POM	Oral	75–300 mg bd	Dose titration required License for neuropathic pain of peripheral origin	Pancreatitis; abnormal LFTs
Non-steroidal anti-inflammatory drugs	10.1.1	Ibuprofen	IP/SP	GSL/P/POM	Oral	1.2–1.8 g daily in divided doses		Angioedema; bronchospasm; vertigo; tinnitus
		Diclofenac	IP/SP	POM	Oral	50 mg tds or 75 mg bd (MR preparation)	Acute 50 mg tds only	Angioedema; bronchospasm; vertigo; tinnitus

Source: Used with kind permission of © NUH NHS Trust.

IP, independent prescriber; SP, supplementary prescriber; POM, prescription only medicine; P, pharmacy; CD POM, controlled drug prescription only medicine; CD, controlled drug; GSL, general sales list; PL, product licence; MR, modified release; TCA, tricyclic antidepressant.

- Collates evidence against their job outline;
- Responds to practice developments;
- Participates in mentorship/buddying nurse prescribers post-qualification.

Examples of evidence in their professional portfolios are required for their annual personal development review. The prescriber may participate in local or national clinical audits and report the outcomes in their portfolio along with reflective learning. Prescribing should also include best evidence-based practice according to local and national guidelines.

A review of related critical incidents and reflective learning could be included along with examples of clinical record keeping, medicines monitoring information and advisory letters to GPs. Critical incidents provide excellent opportunities for learning as simple questions such as 'what happened' and 'what caused it to happen' can provide a framework for reflection, which leads to better understanding and ultimately improvement in the processes of care (Tripp 1993). The reduction of medication errors has been the focus of many papers but those taking an critical incident approach reveal some excellent insights into how such processes can ultimately improve care by reducing errors (Cox *et al.* 2001; Woodward 2009). All prescribers are advised to reflect on their practice with a view to potential research and use compliments or complaints from patients or other professionals to identify their personal learning needs and areas for improvement. Group or individual clinical supervision time is regularly included within the pain services working week.

Justifying the advanced nursing contribution to develop nurse prescribing in pain management

My reflection on the 'advanced nursing contribution' is framed by an excellent study undertaken by Molly Courtenay (Stenner & Courtenay 2007) who used a qualitative, with semi-structured interviews of 26 nurses, who treat patients with pain. This study explored how nurses had adopted the role of prescribing and identified how the restrictions on prescribing controlled drugs impacted on practice. The nurses interviewed consisted of clinical nurse specialists in pain (15), nurse consultants (6), Macmillan nurses (2), clinical nurse managers (2) and lead pain nurse (1). Most nurses worked in hospital settings (21), with 5 in community settings. The four themes which make up the findings frame my own reflections and are discussed below.

The theme 'context' of pain management includes difficulties related to outpatient prescriptions for patients, which were not encouraged due to budgetary controls. This reflects my own experiences as the trust encouraged all clinicians to use outpatient prescription advice yellow forms to be given to the GPs, resulting in the cost of the medication being covered by primary care, not the hospital. Legislative restrictions caused confusion and ambiguity for prescribers, e.g. for the management of post-operative pain and the prescribing of morphine, how long is the post-operative period, 1 week, 2 weeks, 6 months? Two patients could be on the same ward and one patient experiencing severe pain pre-operatively and another patient in pain post-operatively.

The nurse can prescribe analgesia for the former but not the latter. Similarly, a patient experiencing chronic degenerative pain cannot be prescribed morphine by non-medical prescribers, as the condition is not considered to be degenerating towards death. Palliative care and long-term chronic disease management are quite blurred, leading to inequality for patients.

The second theme from Courtenay's study was 'Teams and Relationships' and again this reflected my experiences where there was a lack of medical staff understanding of nurse prescribing and the knowledge base required. This can create a barrier as staff are not working seamlessly across boundaries as they do not understand each other's roles and responsibilities. This ultimately does not maximise opportunities for good team work and communication and requires a dedicated effort to continually provide education and information about these roles.

A further theme of 'autonomy' relates to where nurses working in acute pain services gave examples of faster access to treatment for patients, e.g. prior to the prescribing qualification, the nurse-advised medications, but the following day the advice had not been acted upon. Delays of 24 hours for the patients were common. Nurses supplementary prescribing for patients in chronic pain services gave examples of improvements in patient information, education and prescribing of controlled drugs.

Finally, a 'supportive environment' was highlighted with examples of supportive clinicians, regular clinical supervision, peer support, professional networks and nurses involved with policy development. In our integrated pain service we arranged a weekly group clinical supervision session over a lunchtime. Multiprofessionals, a consultant anaesthetist, pharmacist, nurse specialists and visiting learners to the department brought difficult 'pain problems for patients' to the group session for discussion and formulation of an evidence-based treatment plan.

Nurses who undertake the role of prescriber and work with people experiencing pain experience many barriers in their endeavour to provide good pain management. Finding ways to overcome these challenges and improve care is central to those advancing practice. This section has illustrated several initiatives which have attempted to overcome these difficulties by working across boundaries and demonstrating practice at this level.

Conclusions

Leadership and management should ensure a clarity on responsibilities, with clinical teams working together, such as described by the multiprofessional NMPAS group working together to develop a trust policy. Patient safety remains paramount with adverse incidents reported and systems in place for trusts to learn from these and make the necessary improvements (Healthcare Commission 2008). The dynamic improvements to legislation included a consultation exercise to expand the number of controlled drugs nurses are able to prescribe independently. This includes a variety of options for nurses to prescribe any controlled drug within their area of competence. This potentially will contribute to further improvements in the patients' experiences, e.g. all patients in severe acute pain (not just post-operative patients) will be able to have strong opiates prescribed. There are occasions when morphine is not the most appropriate strong opiate to be prescribed for some patients. Nurse specialists may be able to consider oxycodone or Fentanyl transdermal patches.

Non-medical prescribing for patients with acute or chronic pain has the potential to ignite vast improvements in the management of pain, either in hospital or community settings. Multimodal analgesia improves pain relief and can reduce the incidence and severity of side effects from other drugs. For example, prescribing paracetamol concurrently with opiates can significantly reduce the need for high-dose opiates. Nurse specialists with advanced knowledge and skills are able to prescribe analgesics based on the assessment of pain, its intensity and nature, as recommended by the WHO: where possible by the mouth, by the clock, by the ladder. Timely prescriptions and administration of analgesics can improve pain relief and may reduce morbidity and mortality. Advanced knowledge and understanding of the mechanisms and risks of particular analgesic treatments will improve the safety and effectiveness of prescribing. Local guidelines can be tailored to the individual patient needs, together with adequate education of other professionals, patients and their carers.

References

Bach, M., 2007. Changing environment for opioid prescribing. Combatting the stigma around opioid analgesics. *Pain Europe*, 6(4), 6.

Baird, A., 2005. Independent and supplementary prescribing and PGDs. *Nursing Standard*, 19(51), 51–56.

Bence, A., 2008. Back to the future? *NMC news*, (Feb. No.23), 10–13.

Bennett, O., 2005. *Unpublished MSc Improving Pain Management on Medical Wards*. Nottingham: Nottingham University Hospital.

British Pain Society, 2004. *Recommendations for the Appropriate Use of Opioids in Persistent Non-Cancer Pain*. London: British Pain Society.

Chung, J., Lui, J.C., 2003. Postoperative pain management: study of patients' level of pain and satisfaction with health care providers' responsiveness to their reports of pain. *Nursing and Health Sciences*, 5(1), 13–18.

Courtenay, M., Griffiths, M., 2006. Non-medical prescribing: an overview. In Courtenay, M., Griffiths, M., (eds), *Independent and Supplement Prescribing, An Essential Guide*, pp. 1–6. Cambridge: Cambridge University Press.

Cox, P., D'Amato, S., Tillotson, D., 2001. Reducing medication errors. *American Journal of Medical Quality* [serial online]. 16(3), 81–86. Available at CINAHL Database with full text, Ipswich, MA [accessed 11 May 2009].

Darzi, L., 2007. *Our NHS Our Future: NHS Next Stage Review – Interim Report*. London: Department of Health.

Department of Health, 1989. *Report of the Advisory Group on Nurse Prescribing* (1st Crown Report). London: DH.

Department of Health, 1999. *Review of the Prescribing, Supply and Administration of Medicines* (2nd Crown Report). London: DH.

Department of Health, 2000a. *Health Service Circular, Patient Group Directions [England Only]*. London: NHS Executive Department of Health, HSC 2000/026.

Department of Health, 2000b. *The NHS Plan: A Plan for Investment, A Plan for Reform*. London: DH.

Department of Health, 2003. *Supplementary Prescribing By Nurses and Pharmacists within the NHS in England: A Guide for Implementation.* London: DH.

Department of Health, 2005. *Supplementary Prescribing by Nurses, Pharmacists, Chiropodists/Podiatrists, Physiotherapists and Radiographers within the NHS in England.* London: DH.

Department of Health, 2006a. *Improving Patients Access to Medicines: A Guide to Implementing Nurse and Pharmacist Independent Prescribing within the NHS in England.* London: DH.

Department of Health, 2006b. *Safer Management of Controlled Drugs (CDs): Private CD Prescriptions and Other Changes to the Prescribing and Dispensing of Controlled Drugs (CDs).* Guidance for Implementation. June. Final Guideline. London: DH.

Department of Health and Social Security, 1986. *Neighbourhood Nursing: A Focus for Care* (Cumberlege Report). London: DHSS.

Fagerhaugh, S.Y., Strauss, A., 1977. *Politics of Pain Management: Staff-Patient Interaction.* London: Addison-Wesley.

Gregory, J., Bramwell, J., 2008. Enabling nurses to administer timely pain relief. *Journal of the Pain Network UK*, 10(7), 8–9.

Healthcare Commission, 2008. Inspecting informing improving. Available at www.cqc.org.uk [accessed 11 May 2009].

Jones, M., 2004. Nurse prescribing: a case study in policy influence. *Journal of Nursing Management*, 12, 266–272.

Jordan, S., Griffiths, H., 2004. Nurse prescribing: developing the evaluation agenda. *Nursing Standard*, 18(29), 40–44.

Marks, R., Sachar, E., 1973. The under treatment of medical inpatients with narcotic analgesics. *Annals of Internal Medicine*, 78, 173–181.

McHale, J., 2003. A review of the legal framework for accountable nurse prescribing. *Nurse Prescribing*, 1(3), 107–112.

National Prescribing Centre, 2001. *Maintaining Competency in Prescribing. An Outline Framework to Help Nurse Prescribers*, 1st edn. Liverpool: NPC.

National Prescribing Centre, 2003. *Supplementary Prescribing. A Resource to Help Healthcare Professionals to Understand the Framework and Opportunities.* Liverpool: NPC.

NUH-NMPAS (Nottingham University Hospitals), 2007. *Operational Policy for the Prescribing of Medicines by Non-Medical Prescribers.* Nottingham: NMPAS.

Picker Institute Europe, 2002, 2004. *National Patient Surveys.* London: Picker Institute. Available at http://www.pickereurope.org/publications [accessed 11 May 2009].

Stenner, K., Courtenay, M., 2008. The role of interprofessional relationships and support for nurse prescribing in acute and chronic pain. *Journal of Advanced Nursing*, 63(3), 276–283.

Svensson, I., Sjöström, B., Haljamäe, H., 2000. Assessment of pain experiences after elective surgery. *Journal of Pain and Symptom Management*, 20(3), 193–201.

Tripp, D., 1993. *Critical Incidents in Teaching: Developing Professional Judgement.* London: Routledge.

VanDenKerkhof, E., Goldstein, D., 2004. The prevalence of chronic postsurgical pain in Canada. *Canadian Journal of Anaesthesia*, 51, A20.

Warner, D., 2005. Theory of nurse prescribing. *Journal of Community Nursing*, 19(4), 12–16.

Woodward, S., 2009. On the key role of nurses in incident reporting. *Nursing Times* [serial online]. 105(9), 27–27. Available at British Nursing Index Database, Ipswich, MA [accessed 11 May 2009].

Chapter 11
Nurses leading the development of interprofessional education in pain management

Ann Taylor

Introduction

This chapter examines the rationale and development of an interprofesional pain education course initially to address local need but subsequently leading to the development of the world's first interprofessional, distance learning diploma and MSc in pain management in 1996 at Cardiff University. It describes the major events which created the impetus to develop an interprofessional master's in pain management course.

Interprofessional education (IPE) has been defined as occurring:

> When two or more professions learn with, from and about each other to improve the collaboration and the quality of care (CAIPE 2002).

IPE has a central role in the NHS and requires health professionals to be prepared for interprofessional working (Finch 2000). As health care changes to deal with the demands of society, differing global public health concerns, an aging population and an increased emphasis on long-term management of chronic illness, the delivery of care by a range of professionals who can cooperate in the best interest of the patient is essential (Wood 2001).

Health professionals from many disciplines need to work together effectively to address the multidimensional nature of pain when managing patients with complex problems and their carers and significant others. This is an important issue and illustrated by the way the MSc programme and other strategic documents I have been involved with have been structured. The MSc and the *Service Redevelopment and Commissioning Directives for Chronic Non-Malignant Pain* in Wales (Taylor 2008) both promote good multiprofessional working, and structures are in place to enhance IPE.

Although each professional will have his or her own focus, there are shared goals and outcomes that the team will need to work together to achieve. Therefore, it would seem logical that all of us have the opportunity to be educated with and experience the work of other professionals involved in pain management. This permits understanding of the roles of other professional groups, facilitates working with other professionals in the context of a team and supports the organisation in providing flexibility in career routes (Finch 2000).

Historically, pain has been poorly assessed and managed and it was not until the Working Party Report of the Royal College of Surgeons and then College of Anaesthetists (1990) that major changes were proposed to address pain after surgery, including the promotion of adequate levels of education for all involved in the care of patients in pain.

Prior to the Working Party Report (Royal College of Surgeons and College of Anaesthetists 1990), during the late 1980s, I noticed, as a member of the intensive care team, that a number of patients were admitted with chest infections, resulting from acute post-operative pain. It appeared that analgesia was either not prescribed or has been withheld because ward staff believed that opioid side effects would result in patients being unable to breath and cough adequately and there appeared to be little understanding that not giving analgesia resulted in a similar outcome. At this time, Professor Bridget Dimond (author of legal health care texts) was leading a series of forums to discuss patients' rights and responsibilities and on attending these, I spoke about patients' rights to have good pain relief and she challenged me to do something about this. It was a difficult challenge because acute post-operative pain was not a priority and there was little published evidence or champions trying to address good pain management.

I also was in the process of conducting some course-related research within what was then the largest accident and emergency (A&E) department in Wales and one of the largest in the UK. This illuminated several issues for pain education, notably poor judgements made by the staff, poor levels of communication and lack of rigorous assessment. For instance, a prostitute who had extremely painful pelvic inflammatory disease was not offered any analgesia but a young rugby player was; a combatative and noisy patient with Alzheimer's disease and a fractured neck of femur had analgesia, but the withdrawn patient also suffering from Alzheimer's disease had no analgesia as she was not perceived to be in any pain. Junior doctors did not prescribe analgesia in the mistaken belief that the consultants did not like analgesia being prescribed until they had seen the patient and the consultants assumed that analgesia had been given. It was not that the staff were uncaring; they had little knowledge, though their actions were in the best interest of the patient (if the prostitute experienced severe pain, it may prevent her from returning to that role when better). It became clear from clinical practice and research observation that within the hospital there was a lack of knowledge about pain assessment and management, poor communication between senior health care professionals and junior staff, and poor team working.

Pain is a multidimensional phenomenon that involves a biopsychosocial perspective, and it therefore made sense to me that a range of health professions would need to work interprofessionally to address pain management satisfactorily. Nurses needed to assess pain and to be able to offer good analgesia (Haigh 2001), and the medical staff needed to prescribe adequately. This led to a series of monthly pain days which were interprofessional and attempted to provide an evidence base to improve care. They also had the added benefit of allowing staff to share their experiences, sometimes in a heated way, but with careful chairing the groups were moved away from blaming each other for inadequacies and towards accepting joint responsibility for doing it right.

I attempted to introduce regular pain assessment in the wards and in A&E. This was a clinically driven initiative and although pain was not recognised as important by my senior nursing colleagues, I had great support from my senior medical colleagues who ran the intensive care unit. There was a great deal of reticence with nurses to assess pain; they did not have the time and if they did have the time, the pain relief they could offer was inadequate. Nurses felt it only raised patients' expectations, and nurses felt powerless to address these. Doctors were reluctant to prescribe regular, strong analgesia because of fears and misconceptions and there was little in the way of good practice initiatives to use to illustrate what should be undertaken. Similar problems were identified in an article by Helen Taylor (1997), a previous MSc student, who also implemented pain assessment in a district general hospital. I had to draw on my medical colleagues to insist that pain assessment, education and appropriate management were going to be driven through.

I wrote a letter to the Women's Royal Voluntary Service asking if they would purchase some patient-controlled analgesia (PCA) machines for the hospital, and between their contribution and the hospital management, 12 devices were made available. Nurses began to assess pain more regularly in order to ensure that patients were safely managed and realised that if the pain was better managed, patients could do more themselves. Therefore, nursing time could be reinvested in pain assessment and good management. An acute pain service was started in the late 1980s operating on 'good will' as there was no dedicated staff and those involved could only donate time when the intensive care unit was not busy. Eventually, my medical colleagues made it part of their working day and after dealing with the critically ill patients, they did a pain round in the hospital visiting patients on PCA and those receiving epidural analgesia.

I then obtained a secondment which involved establishing a number of acute pain services across Wales and working with existing acute pain services. Similar to the local issues discussed previously, the drivers for interprofessional pain education came from poor communication, lack of accountability and responsibility for pain management, and poor team working. Educational initiatives needed to address these issues and involve professionals responsible for managing pain.

From experiences gained locally and through talking to people involved in pain management, it became clear that there was a need for formal pain education. I reflected on what clinicians would want to know, how best to deliver education to clinicians who may be single-handed practitioners and/or could not take regular time of work and how to ensure that the course was interprofessional. By chance, I met an Open University tutor and discussed my ideas with him; he suggested a distance learning format. I discussed my ideas with the then Director of the School of Nursing, who, unfortunately, was not supportive and so took my ideas to Professor Rosen and Professor Vickers (the Cardiff Palliator inventors – the first patient-controlled analgesic pump) and they were keen to help. I negotiated a role and some funding in order to set up, validate and run the first interprofessional, distance learning diploma in pain management in 1994 and undertook commercial research to pump prime my salary. The course was revalidated to fulfil MSc level learning outcomes, and in 1996, the first MSc in pain management was launched in Cardiff.

To evaluate the effectiveness of IPE, Irajpour (2006) undertook a systematic review of four studies, two randomised controlled studies and two quasi-experimental studies. The outcome was inconclusive and no clear answer to the question of whether IPE is effective in pain management could be reached. Zwarenstein *et al.* (2001) concluded in a *Cochrane Database of Systematic Reviews* that despite finding a large body of literature on the evaluation of IPE, studies lacked the methodological rigour needed to begin to convincingly understand the impact of IPE on professional practice and/or health care outcomes. Much of the published work on outcomes of IPE relies on the perceptions and subjective responses of those who have been through an IPE programme with little available research on patient outcomes, changes to organisational practice and changes in individual behaviour (Freeth *et al.* 2005). Therefore, while more evidence is needed to ascertain whether IPE is effective in changing behaviours of health professionals and improving outcomes for patients, this should not be seen as lack of effectiveness.

Developing a formal educational qualification in pain

As indicated above, the aim was to offer an interprofessional, distance learning course in pain management. The course was to be and remains grounded in adult learning philosophy (see Table 11.1) because of the participants we attract (40% senior medical practitioners, 40% senior nurses and 20% professionals allied to medicine). At the time, there was no real perceived need for a formal qualification in pain. The NHS did not require it as a qualification for those involved in pain management nor did professional bodies. In the early 1990s, health care was beginning, albeit slowly, to respond to the Working Party Report but pain management had not developed into the specialism it has today. It highlighted the fact that there should be a need, that clinicians working with people in pain should have a course focused on their needs, providing academic and evidence-based support and the opportunity to network with like-minded health care professionals. It was when we advertised and received a large number of applications it became clear that there was a need.

The course aimed (and still does) to provide the student with the opportunity to explore pain as a multidimensional phenomenon and is underpinned by the International Association for the Study of Pain (IASP) Core Curriculum.

The course has undergone major amendments over 12 years with the adoption of e-learning and the opportunity to be more proactive in engaging the student and allowing the student to plot a pathway through the course. The modules offered include:

(1) evidence-based practice, research and statistics
(2) biopsychosocial approach to pain management
(3) fundamentals in pain management
(4) professional options
(5) management options
(6) case study options

Table 11.1 Key principles in adult learning

Adult learning philosophy	Example of curriculum considerations
Adults are autonomous and self-directed. They need to be free to direct themselves	Options modules and flexibility built into assignment questions
Adults have accumulated a foundation of life experiences and knowledge and they need to connect learning to this knowledge/experience base	Avoiding lectures and the use of group work, problem-based learning, debates and reflective practice centred around case studies
Adults are goal orientates; they usually know what goal they want to attain and therefore appreciate an educational programme that is organised and has clearly defined elements	Facilitating the development of individual aims and objectives and supporting students to realise these within the course; detailed handbook and modularised
Adults are relevancy orientated, learning has to be applicable to their work or other responsibilities of value to them	Linking the educational material to clinical practice and using key clinicians to write material, facilitate workshops, etc., and mark assignments
Adults are practical, focusing on the aspects of a lesson most useful to them in their work	Student-based sessions, reflective exercises and sharing best practice built into the course materials
Adults need to be shown respect	Treating students as partners in their learning, allowing them a voice and respecting their opinions

Source: Adapted from Knowles *et al.* (1984).

I was fortunate to work with people who wanted me to succeed but there were others who had to be persuaded. I did not have much in the way of credibility at the time. I think being dedicated, passionate and motivated to make changes persuaded some, others responded because I kept nagging them (in subtle ways) and unfortunately some were never persuaded. I developed a business plan and persuaded Professors Rosen and Vickers to employ me and believe in the course and the then Chief Nurse of Wales to pump prime some of the course developments. I undertook an honorary acute pain service role in order to have peer support and to gain a sense of belonging and for the contribution I made to the team, they responded by helping and supporting the course. Similarly, I worked within the Chronic Pain Clinic and obtained support and help from the consultants in chronic pain. These experiences improved my credibility.

Developing a planning team which reflected the ethos of the course was essential; it needed to be clinically relevant and interprofessional. To help the process, some of the change theories were useful in getting me to reflect on resources and facilitate the planning process. I wanted the course to be grounded in adult learning philosophy and used Knowles' (1990) characteristics of a creative leader to help introduce the new course. I did not (and probably still do not) really see myself as a creative leader, more a creative facilitator.

The course planning team had representation from all the main professions managing patients in pain and the modules were written by one or two main authors and then critically read and commented on by a range of professionals to ensure that the modules reflected the interprofessional nature of the course: learning from and about each other. Those who were important to my early development and whom I had worked with within intensive care were asked to join the course planning team. Through attending a national conference, I established more help and support for this team and also asked advice from key people within the pain arena as to who would be of value to be on the team.

Accrediting a course to obtain approval is not an easy process. There are many hurdles and as a novice educationalist, it was sometimes difficult to know how much or how little detail was needed in completing the forms and documentation that accompanied this proposal. Persuading University of Wales College of Medicine that there would be a market was also problematic; had a survey been undertaken, this would have alerted potential competitors that this may be an untapped market. An advisory board was held and this provided the team with advice and suggested changes before a formal approval board. Module content, hours of study, aims, objectives and learning outcomes linked to the assessment, all had to be available and were thoroughly scrutinised. After some minor amendments, we obtained approval.

The first diploma course commenced in 1994 with about 40 students and after two further intakes, the course was redesigned to fulfil MSc level and the first MSc in pain management commenced in 1996. Given that my postgraduate qualifications to date had been in nursing, I decided to enrol on the MSc in medical education in 1994 to inform the development of the MSc in pain management. The course has had an intake every year since its inceptions despite competition from other institutions, many of whom have emulated this model. The course is evaluated formally and informally at regular intervals through the use of anonymised questionnaires and the student representative. Student feedback is invaluable and has continuously shaped the course development. Many successful students have returned and are part of the faculty and involved in writing modules, marking and facilitating sessions at the residential weekends.

The interprofessional aspects of the course are extremely important. The modules provide students with the ability to learn from and about other professionals having been authored and critically read by a range of different professionals. They are written in the style of a tutorial with emphasis on using the best available evidence. Residential weekends provide an opportunity for students to meet and this has been evaluated as important for students as they learn from each other and obtain a good network of clinical support. The majority of students undertaking this course are experienced, senior health care professionals. These sessions provide students with an opportunity to interact and deliberate issues in clinical practice. Many work with minimal or no support and have little in the way of recourse to other experts in similar fields, so this provides some clinical support for the students. It also helps improve interprofessional working, group working and communication and networking, as well as presentation skills. The sessions at the residential weekend are facilitated by experts in the field and represent the various professions involved in pain management. They are structured to allow for debate, case study presentations, critical incidence discussions and good practice reviews.

Each distance learning module has an accompanying assessment which facilitates individuals from different professions and specialist areas to consider issues and apply evidence gained to practice. The assignment questions are very broad based and non-specific with the aim of:

- Developing a critical approach to pain management in their health setting involving analysis, reflection, synthesis and evaluation of the literature;
- Challenging traditional approaches to conceptualising pain;
- Challenging traditional treatments regarding pain;
- Reflecting on how the knowledge gained can inform clinical practice.

Assignments are structured to assess higher levels of cognitive function which includes application, analysis and reflection (Curzon 1990; Quinn 1995). Assessments are designed in order to provide the candidate with a chance to demonstrate how he or she frames problems, appraises and replies to alternative views, evaluates evidence and defends conclusions. This is achieved through literature reviews, debates, discussion groups, PowerPoint presentations and other e-learning modalities that we are currently piloting. These skills are needed to assess the quality of literature and assess if it is appropriate to implement change based on research findings and/or expert opinion; one of the course aims at master's level.

Challenges in establishing and managing an interprofessional course

There were numerous challenges in setting up and running the interprofessional courses. Some of the issues have already been raised and others will briefly be addressed.

Developing the business plan for the diploma course was challenging but important. With finite resources, some pump priming and the commercial study money, it was important to budget carefully. Unfortunately, having never completed one previously, and having little idea of exact costs, it was a bit of a disaster (see Table 11.2). It is important, with any new venture to obtain help and support to put together a rigorous business plan and in hindsight I should have obtained help from a health economists and/or a business manager. Recruiting adequate numbers to maintain course viability is always a concern but has never been a real challenge as we attract large numbers on a yearly basis. Several improvements have enhanced the attractiveness of the course, moving toward e-learning, reducing residential components, more online activities, less emphasis on the written assignment and a shorter course. We believe these changes will increase our market share.

An essential aspect of creating an academic course, affiliated with an institution of higher education, was the process of accreditation and validation. The accrediting board needed marketing information to persuade them that no other courses existed and this was to be the first of its kind. The academic credibility was not a problem; the boards were satisfied with the documentation, learning outcomes, use of the IASP curriculum, etc., their concerns revolved around the market. Establishing the market need was difficult; had we sent out questionnaires, then other universities might have

Table 11.2 Considerations when costing a course

Cost	Considerations
Module authors	What rate to pay? If you embrace IPE, then all contributors need to be paid equally and the modules were co-authored by a number of professionals which is costly
Critical readers	These ended up writing a great deal of the modules they critically read and so this increased their fees
Contributors to residential weekends	A fee was built into the cost of the course but as we use national experts, travelling and accommodation were initially not factored in
Computers, printers and office equipment	The existing equipment was old and did not last long, and new equipment was not considered in planning
Staff	Had no budget for extra staff, so for 2 years existed without a secretary or any other team members – had I realised, I could have obtained pump priming if I had put a business case together
Conferences and travel	Needed to ensure that the course was evidence based and up to date and yet did not allow for conference attendance etc., luckily managed to get quite a bit funded from other sources
Stationary, paper, posting, etc.	Assumed that we could use hospital and university provisions but had not realised the huge amount we would require and so quite quickly we had to resource this ourselves

been alerted to our intentions and start the process of validating a similar type course. The Head of Department accepted financial responsibility if the course failed to generate income. This was very stressful at the time, the budget was limited and I had a large team of interested, but unfunded, parties working on the course. The core belief that it would be the first course of its kind was the main encouragement. Fortunately, the first intake was large enough to generate a healthy profit and subsequent intakes followed.

The attitudes of individuals on the course were important to its success. Stereotyping can cloud progress in terms of IPE. For instance, non-medical professionals have found it intimidating to be on courses with medical staff, and medical staff sometimes felt isolated because non-medical staff have not involved them. Much of this is due to poor communication and once the group is aware that despite the professional background, most have similar anxieties and fears, interprofessional interaction and learning improves.

For distance learning courses, it is essential to engage students' interests and teach effectively. Failure as experienced by many distance learning students (usually adult, part-time and fee paying) is viewed as a devastating personal failure, wasted investment of time and money or a 'con' depending on the student (Chambers 1995). Not only is there psychological and social upset for the student, but reactions can damage the course and lead it to be discredited. Distance learning has suffered in the past from the view that it is second best or a quick and easy way to get a qualification (Chambers 1995). Therefore, one of the big challenges was to ensure that the course was fit for purpose and that students could engage with the course material and access appropriate help and advice from the course team. Regular evaluation and the robust way the modules were developed, written and edited as tutorial in print documents with recommended text and self-assessed exercises helped to address the above concerns. Now, the course is well known and few students enter it with unrealistic expectations.

A further challenge, in the health care literature, relates to a lack of evidence supporting professionals' ability to learn interprofessional team skills without having formal education (Hall & Weaver 2001). Little formal education on interprofessional team skills per se was undertaken. Initially, we did undertake some exercises but they were not well evaluated and students felt it more appropriate for them to experience interprofessional team working within the educational sessions relating to pain management. Some of the ways we addressed this were to ask students to bring case studies to share and debate how best to manage the complex scenarios and used role-play to identify key personnel within the groups. Debriefing was important following these sessions as sometimes they became quite heated. We also used critical incidents from practice to get students to reflect on roles and relationships and why, in the absence of good team working, these incidences occurred.

Initially there were challenges in regard to each others' roles, especially the traditional stereotypical ones. For instance, it was expected during group work that the doctor in the group would lead that group and/or provide feedback for the group. Careful facilitation from a range of professionals' expert in either pain management and/or IPE ensured that all students had an opportunity to lead, feedback and participate, that those who felt less confident were supported and helped and that the groups moved away from blame.

A further challenge has been to ensure that with the large numbers of students (about 40–50 students per cohort), there is a sufficient faculty to support them. We now have a large database of successful alumni, many returning as faculty, and offer an induction programme for markers and supervisors. This has also helped in restructuring the curriculum and the material given to students in ensuring that it fulfils the needs of a range of students from a ward nurse wanting to specialise in pain through to an experienced consultant anaesthetist.

Evaluation and the use of audit

The purpose of evaluation for the course was to:

- Establish that the course was providing clinically relevant, research based, up-to-date information for those practising in pain management;
- Explore whether the students thought the course was appropriate for their needs, pitched at the right academic level, kept them motivated and was enjoyable, etc.;
- Ensure that the course had a high academic standard and the students were challenged by the module assignments;
- Ensure that the course met the requirements set out by the validating bodies.

Evaluation has been the area of greatest controversy and weakest technology in all of education, especially in adult education and training (Brookfield 1996). The course planning team wanted the evaluation strategy to rely on student opinion of the value of the course rather than grades awarded to prove success. It was deemed more important to evaluate the worth of the course in relation to informing practice than to evaluate it in terms of grades awarded.

Evaluating the course in terms of patient outcomes, changes in professional's behaviour and in terms of changes in service provision provides is extremely challenging and has been one reported to be one of the outcomes of successful IPE rich data to tailor course direction. However, these data need to be interpreted with some caution. Students come from diverse backgrounds, from different professions and differing levels of expertise and impact they have on their clinical setting. Therefore, evaluation of the above can only be through asking students what they perceive to have happened as a result of them undertaking the course, and this may be coloured by the fact they have invested time and money in undertaking the MSc.

Through formal and informal evaluation, it is clear that the majority of students have learned a wealth of knowledge that has been of practical use and that the course has been seen as highly successful across students with a variety of academic abilities. Students starting the course are asked to write down their aims and objectives, which are revisited at the end of each year to see how the course has helped (or not) the students to meet their aims and objectives.

Questionnaires are used to evaluate the course, one advantage being that it catered for the number of students involved and the distance learning aspect made it difficult to use other techniques. The residential component, the module content, the support given by the course team, as well as global evaluations are requested from students. A combination of closed and open questions were used as there was the potential of getting much richer data that reflected students' needs and interests rather than what the course committee thought students' needs and interests were (Schweibert *et al.* 1996). Quantitative and qualitative data are collected and feed into the quality assurance mechanisms.

The modules are evaluated by a panel of experts used by the course team, who were not necessarily educators as suggested by Holmberg (1996). They included an ethicist, a clinical specialist in the module subject, a potential student, an educationalist, a layperson and an ex-Open University tutor. The panel had a list of questions regarding clinical relevance, evidence-based practice, readability, ability to engage the student flexibility to allow students to self-direct where possible, accuracy of content and level of academic pursuit. It proved a useful exercise to evaluate the modules but neglected the whole learning experience proved costly in terms of time and money. For later modules this was abandoned, and critical reading by professionals other than the authors ensured the modules were interprofessional, evidence based, clinically relevant and up to date.

As part of my own studies for a master's degree I undertook a phenomenological study examining the experiences of female nurses undertaking the course. This also helped to evaluate the impact of the course but obviously within a narrow perspective. From the analysis, five themes emerged which described their journeys through the course. These ranged from experiencing anxiety at the start of course, moving towards helping each other, moving away from group support to focus on educational processes for master's study and independence. The final theme is particularly relevant as it illuminates the transition to master's level, as psychological, social and professional growth was evident. The nurses were able to construct knowledge based on what they had gained from the course and their own intuitions in order to make sense of themselves and their practice. All the nurses spoke of being more mature and having improved self-esteem and all described instances where they no longer had to rely on external validation for their self-identity. The nurses spoke of the knowledge they had constructed in providing them with an improved ability to care and described the continued use of frameworks to underpin practice. These frameworks were constructed by the nurses and were based upon their experiences and knowledge of interprofessional pain management, and they felt more satisfied in their clinical roles. The nurses now perceived themselves as being part of a team rather than outside it; they felt valued, respected and capable. The nurses spoke of making connections that helped tie together pockets of knowledge and spoke of understanding that all knowledge was relative. The nurses wanted nursing to be seen as important in the care of patients in pain and spoke of making a difference; they now wanted to be respected for being nurses. Armed with the academic knowledge, confidence and self-worth, they provided examples of how they impacted on the care of patients in pain.

Evaluation of education programmes is important for continued improvement and learning. My own study illustrated a new and relatively unexplored perspective of growth and change experienced by female nurses studying this course. By focusing on a subgroup it added a unique viewpoint which gave insight into the transitions made during this journey.

Justifying the advanced nursing contribution

The advanced contribution pertains to the leadership and vision that I gave to the development of the course. I feel that I crossed traditional boundaries and made connections. Importantly I saw the need for IPE and felt comfortable taking this forward. The MSc in medical education helped me to think more laterally about solving the problem of engaging and supporting adult learners who were also senior health professionals. It also gave the confidence to take forward the major changes we recently have obtained approval for. In defining an 'advanced nursing contribution', may be a higher level degree is important in this. In justifying an advanced nursing contribution, it has made me reflect on whether the outcome, i.e. a successful interprofessional MSc in pain management, is partly due to me being a nurse or partly due to being who I am. Did it take a nurse to do what I have done? Could it equally have been a doctor, physiotherapist, psychologist, etc.? As a nurse working within ICU, I was used to working within an interprofessional team that in the main was built on trust and respect and therefore, it may have been this nursing experience that contributed to my desire to make the planned course an interprofessional one.

As a nurse, I had undertaken a variety of academic courses that allowed me to consider topics that I feel are important in delivering and managing IPE. These included communication, counselling, team working and empathy. They gave me the credibility to engage with others and persuade them for the need for the MSc in pain management. My knowledge helped me to understand why students may react in the way that they do, helped me to diffuse difficult and confrontational situations and support stressed, anxious and grieving individuals during their educational experience. Again, other professionals have such skills and so it would be difficult to state that they were nurse specific.

Nurses have skills in being conduits of information for various team members involved in patient care and I do feel that nurses have a better sight of the 'bigger picture' and also have more idea of the role of different professions. This helped me in identifying who should be involved in the course and how to structure it. Undertaking the MSc in medical education was useful as it allowed me to step out of traditional nursing academic courses and experience the learning environment of another professional.

The achievements I have made have not been in a vacuum; I have had a great deal of help and support from a range of professionals. The role I took on in developing and managing an IPE, distance learning course, MSc in pain management was a new one to me. It was advanced at the time as my role was outside the traditional one of nurse tutor in a School of Nursing. I had little formal educational qualifications and a steep learning curve in addressing the knowledge deficits in terms of education. The skills utilised in planning, delivering and managing the curriculum are, I feel, advanced ones. I developed them through my experiences as a nurse. In fact, the themes generated in my phenomenological study reflect my transition from that of a course organiser to that of a senior lecturer over the years.

Conclusions

The course has been incredibly successful and a large number (approximately 700 health care professionals) of students have successfully completed the certificate, diploma and MSc options. The course attracts students from all over the world. It has a national and international reputation and many alumni recommend their colleagues to attend.

How the course impacts on clinical practice is impossible to say and research is required to explore this further. Now I have a team of lecturers who can take responsibility for leading the courses that we run, this will give me time to undertake some pedagogical research.

A great deal of thought went into ensuring that the course is bespoke to the needs of the students and all material has been written with clinicians working with people in pain in mind. The curriculum has been considered from an interprofessional perspective with major opportunities available to network and learn from and about other professionals. Previous students who want to return and become part of the faculty are encouraged to do so as these are now senior pain management clinicians and their input adds credibility to the course. The course has been updated regularly to respond to the ever-increasing evidence base and NHS initiatives.

Following the success of the course, a number of other MSc courses developed across the UK and further a field. To ensure we have a competitive edge, the course is now undergoing major revisions to exploit the full potential of e-learning. We have an e-learning technician employed and materials will be crafted so that the student's experience is enhanced through a range of different approaches to learning and assessment. The development and success of a pain management course, such as this, reflects an exemplar of how advanced knowledge in education can be channelled to a successful outcome. My role as a nurse and my initial experiences shaped this development and whilst the outcome is interprofessional, it would not have been achieved without the ethos and philosophy underpinned by nursing.

References

Brookfield, S.D., 1996. *Understanding and Facilitating Adult Learning*. Milton Keynes: Open University Press.

Centre for the Advancement of Interprofessional Education (CAIPE), 2002. Defining IPE. Available at http://www.caipe.org.uk/about-us/defining-ipe/ [accessed 10 February 2009].

Chambers, E., 1995. Course evaluation and academic quality. In Lockwood, F. (ed.), *Open and Distance Learning Today*, 1st edn, pp. 343–353. London: Routledge Press.

Curzon, L.B., 1990. *Teaching in Further Education*, 4th edn. London: Cassell.

Finch, J., 2000. Interprofessional education and team working: a view from the education providers. *BMJ*, 321, 1138–1140.

Freeth, D., Reeves, S., Koppel, I., Hammick, M., Barr, H., 2005. *Evaluation Interprofessional Education: A Self-Help Guide*. London: Higher Education Academy.

Haigh, C., 2001. Contribution of a multiprofessional team to pain management. *British Journal Nursing*, 10, 370–374.

Hall, P., Weaver, L., 2001. Interprofessional education and teamwork: a long and winding road. *Medical Education*, 35, 867–875.

Holmberg, B., 1996. *Theory and Practice of Distance Education*. London: Routledge Studies in Distance Education.

Irajpour, A., 2006. Interprofessional education: a facilitator to enhance pain management? *Journal of Interprofessional Care*, 20, 675–678.

Knowles, M., 1990. *The Adult Learner, A Neglected Species*. Houston: Gulf Publishing Company.

Knowles, M., 1984. *Andragogy in Action: Applying Modern Principles of Adult Education*. San Francisco: Jossey Bass.

Quinn, F.M., 1995. *The Principles and Practice of Nurse Education*, 3rd edn. London: Chapman & Hall.

Royal College of Surgeons and College of Anaesthetists, 1990. *Working Party of the Commission on the Provision of Surgical Services. Pain after Surgery*. London: Royal College of Surgeons, College of Anaesthetists.

Schweibert, P., Cacy, D., Davis, A., Crandall, S., 1996. Using narrative student feedback to evaluate the impact of a family medicine clerkship. *Teaching and Learning in Medicine*, 8, 158–163.

Taylor, A.M., 2008. *Service Development and Commissioning Directives: Chronic Non-Malignant Pain*. Cardiff: Welsh Assembly Government.

Taylor, H., 1997. Pain scoring as a formal pain assessment tool. *Nursing Standard*, 11, 40–42.

Wood, D.F., 2001. Interprofessional education – still more questions than answers. *Medical Education*, 35, 816–817.

Zwarenstein, M., Reeves, S., Barr, H., Hammick, M., Koppel, I., Atkins, J., 2001. Interprofessional education: effects on professional practice and health care outcomes. *Cochrane Database of Systematic Reviews*, (1): CD002213.

Chapter 12
New knowledge for advancing practice in pain management

Martin Christensen and Eloise Carr

Introduction

The purpose of this final chapter is to capture the thematic analysis of the contributions to 'advancing practice' embedded in this book. The process for this is briefly described below. We do not intend this to be an in-depth theoretical discussion but rather a pragmatic perspective on the issues we believe, informed by these contributors, to be central to advancing practice in the context of pain management.

At the beginning of this book we offered a description of what constituted advanced and advancing practice in terms of the attributes and knowledge inherent in developing and advancing practice not only in pain management but nursing practice as well. Central to this development is the knowing-how knowing-that framework which conceptualises the knowledge and action seen with clinical decision-making. Within this framework, in particular the knowing-how element, we suggest there are a number of variables which form the knowledge which instructs the knowing-that. For example, the knowing-what is embedded within pattern recognition, knowing-how is derived from practical and experiential learning, and knowing-why is theoretical knowledge, all of which culminates into the knowing-that – the deliberative action based on an extensive understanding of the situation, a trademark provided by the contributors in this book.

Whilst it might not be readily self-evident that these traits are visible within the examples contained in the preceding chapters, this framework serves as an underlying theme of advancement and if questioned further, it would become apparent that these practitioners exhibit these different knowledge strands in a clinical environment. It might well be evident to some readers that this framework has a number of different applications, for example, when developing a knowledge integration model for practice or for mapping knowledge against key competencies such as the Department of Health's (DH's) Knowledge and Skills Framework (DH 2004). In the context of this book we are using it to define the advancing practice of specialist pain practitioners, as they forge the boundaries of nursing practice with many creating roles traditionally seen within the realm of medical practice. We are not, however, suggesting that the vignettes portrayed within this book set a precedent as to what advanced and advancing practice are; moreover, they represent different perspectives as to how these individual practitioners have advanced practice within the sphere of pain management and have crossed those 'blurred' boundaries between nursing, medicine and other health professionals. Admittedly overturning the traditional hierarchical models of care delivery is not easy. Many of the practitioners' narratives provide good examples of interprofessional cooperation and working, in order to develop the service, but more importantly to promote effective patient care and enhance the patient's experience of the health care service.

Emerging themes As described at the outset of this book, the aim of this chapter was to thematically capture key aspects related to the nursing contribution to advancing practice in pain management. This was achieved by reviewing each chapter, and in particular the knowledge contribution and coding key aspects. These were then collapsed to inform three main themes. First, it is the notable presence of independence and entrepreneurship which is evident throughout many aspects of the narratives presented here (especially Chapter 7). Second is the emergence of clinical leadership, as evidenced by crossing boundaries and the development of services, and finally interprofessional working. Whilst it would be ideal to discuss professional independence and entrepreneurship in order to provide insight for others to follow and implement, we have chosen to focus on clinical leadership and interprofessional working which we believe significantly strengthen the premise of advancing and advanced nursing practice. These themes are not surprises as many documents discussing advanced practice, and the required competencies indicate such qualities are essential to the notion of 'advanced' practice (Royal College of Nursing 2003; Por 2008). It is reassuring that these strong themes emerge in these narratives to validate the practitioners endeavours, but we suggest they go further to elucidate practice which moves beyond describing the competencies for advanced practice, and reveal the complexity of working at this level and the uniqueness of each endeavour. They make transparent the journey experienced by these advanced practitioners in the context of pain management.

Clinical leadership

Today's nurse leaders inspire a shared image of clinical practice by instilling a strong sense of direction and vision (Cain 2005; Siriwardena 2006). There is an expectation, of course, that in order to advance practice the leadership qualities that epitomise practice should seen to:

> . . . adjust the boundaries for the development of future practice, pioneering and developing new roles responsive to changing needs . . . advancing clinical practice, research and education to enrich professional practice as a whole. (United Kingdom Central Council 2008)

This could not be more evident in the DH's (2000a) *A Service for All Talents: Developing the NHS Workforce*, where one of the recommendations had a major impact on the nursing career structure: that of establishing specialist and consultant nursing posts. Key to this was the importance placed on attaining higher academic awards, increased professional autonomy and clinical responsibility. However, the term leadership often meant adopting a shared vision and a strong belief value in what was being achieved

Table 12.1   Leadership qualities

Transactional leadership	Clinical leadership
Charisma	Peer credibility
Vision	Clinical expertise
Inspiration	Supportive to the clinical team
Strong belief ethic	Education and research
Impersonal	Motivation and energy
At times solitary	Empathy
	Humanism
	Interpersonal skills

normally from one person. Yet clinical leaders have additional characteristics that often set them apart from the traditional leadership role (see Table 12.1; Siriwardena 2006), the core values seen with nurse consultants and clinical nurse specialists.

This list of what constitutes leadership qualities is not exhaustive; moreover, it would be easy to suggest that the work portrayed in this book demonstrates these core clinical leadership values and in some cases this is clearly noticeable. Take, for example, the setting up of a nurse-led femoral nerve block service. As part of her role, Mandy Layzell (Chapter 2) suggested that:

> As team leader I am responsible for ensuring that the service is run safely. I will provide support and supervision for my colleagues in the team and discuss any issues that are raising concern. I regularly review audit data we collect to ensure that the procedure is performed safely and that patients are benefiting, and progress is disseminated to management and specialist committee members. In addition, I am responsible for ensuring that the relevant documentation is up to date and evidence-based.

Again this is identified in Gillian Chumbley's work (Chapter 3) in developing a nurse-led ketamine service for individuals experiencing acute and chronic post-operative pain. Whilst primarily she discusses the setting up of the service to administer ketamine, there is an underlying theme of clinical leadership:

> To adopt a new method of working into routine practice, it takes an individual who is passionate about the benefits, who has collated the scientific evidence, has recognised a gap in the management of patients and who can identify how the change can be incorporated into current practice. This is made easier if you are known and respected by the organisation. Although the sub-roles of educator, researcher and consultant are the basic requirements to move practice forward, it is essential to be recognised as an experienced expert in your field. An advanced practitioner has to have a working knowledge of the scientific evidence and be comfortable conversing with colleagues, from a range of professions, at this level. For advanced nursing practice to be taken seriously, we have to use the correct language. Higher educational degrees give nurses the confidence, knowledge and skills to recognise, disseminate and utilise robust research.

As exemplified here, the transformational leadership qualities allow engagement in a process, where one or more people connect with each other in a way that elevates leaders and followers to higher levels of motivation and in doing so accelerates progress. The importance of leadership is embedded in the NHS reforms and made explicit in the DH publication (2008) *A High Quality Workforce: NHS Next Stage Review*, which emphasises not only the role of leadership in workforce development but the shift in health care from secondary to primary care. Throughout this book it is evident that a number of new initiatives have been developed and created to drive a new culture of care in which nursing leadership is at the forefront. Many contributors to the book would agree that clinical leadership is an important means of strengthening nursing and establishing effective interprofessional team collaboration, all of which requires adaptability and receptivity to change – the central tenant to the NHS Plan (DH 2000b).

Crossing boundaries and the development of services

Continuing health reforms and health care pressures have meant that traditional medical roles are now being undertaken by suitably trained, educated and competent nurses. Whilst this calls for a greater cooperation between the professions, it is the responsiveness to service user need that is the driving force behind a more streamlined approach to the way care is delivered. Where there are a number of examples within the book that discuss the entrepreneurship associated with developing services, it is evident that key to these developments is the meeting of an unmet need; this is illustrated in the setting up of an acupuncture service (Ruth Heafield and colleagues, Chapter 6):

> The development of any new service requires careful consideration of the political, clinical and governance issues; therefore, advanced skills are required to understand and manage the complexity of issues during negotiation and implementation of such services. The development of an acupuncture service in the current climate requires all these skills and more. The nurse must be aware of the current funding pathways and ensure that the service is sustainable and appropriately placed linking into existing services to serve the best interests of the clients. The educational aspects of staff training and development are crucial for the development and maintenance of the service. This is of particular importance currently as mandatory registration for acupuncture is, as discussed earlier, a hot political debate. Careful consideration must also be taken to identify the potential risks of the service and systems put in place to minimise those risks and record and manage any untoward incidents.

Despite the excellence in meeting unmet needs such as those portrayed above, there is clearly a degree of autonomy present, discussed in this context as the developing of practice but also one's own role, and with this comes development of clinical judgement. We make this connection explicit in Chapter 1, where we suggested that a registered nurse who has acquired the expert knowledge base, complex decision-making skills and clinical competencies for expanded practice is in a position to advance and develop practice. However, it is becoming more prevalent that higher educational awards are paramount in gaining acceptance in these advancing roles; for example:

> For nurses to undertake these clinics some advanced education in pain management would be required and ideally they would need to be a prescriber in primary care to optimise cost–benefit. There are now a significant number of specialist pain nurses who have undergone a degree in this subject and have been closely involved in the care of patients in pain for many years. (Ruth Heafield, Chapter 6)

Therefore, it would seem that in order to advance practice in pain management, achieve a degree of autonomy and be seen to setting new standards of care delivery outside the typical norm, nurses are encouraged to undertake advanced educational courses. In reflecting on the development of a master's programme in pain management, Ann Taylor (Chapter 11) recognised that her own higher level education set the precedent for others to follow. She suggests that:

> I feel that I crossed traditional boundaries and made connections. Importantly I saw the need for IPE and felt comfortable taking this forward. The MSc in medical education helped me to think more laterally about solving the problem of engaging and supporting adult learners who were also senior health professionals. It also gave the confidence to take forward the major changes we recently have obtained approval for. In defining an 'advanced nursing contribution', may be a higher level degree is important in this. In justifying an advanced nursing contribution, it has made me reflect on whether the outcome, i.e. a successful interprofessional MSc in pain management, is partly due to me being a nurse or partly due to being who I am. Did it take a nurse to do what I have done? Could it equally have been a doctor, physiotherapist, psychologist, etc.? As a nurse working within ICU, I was used to working within an interprofessional team that in the main was built on trust and respect and therefore, it may have been this nursing experience that contributed to my desire to make the planned course an interprofessional one.

Ann raises an important issue in that the crossing of boundaries also sets the other exemplars within the book into the context of advancing practice in pain management. This could not be more prominent where individual practitioners in the course of their work are undertaking patient caseloads to offset, in some cases, medical case work and prescribing responsibilities. Therefore, this leads nicely onto interprofessional team working.

Interprofessional working

The focus of the book on nursing does not negate the importance of working effectively within an interprofessional team. Indeed, it is often the ability to do this, which enables the development of the service to flourish. This emergent theme is present in each chapter and we use the term to capture a range of activities, including working effectively within an interprofessional team, working across professional groups and participating in interprofessional education.

Each chapter makes references to the importance of working alongside other health professionals, doctors, physiotherapists, managers, pharmacist, etc.

> Support from the multidisciplinary pain team (nurses, anaesthetists, pharmacists, physiotherapists and psychologists) was fundamental to the evolution and success of the project. (Felicia Cox, Chapter 5)

The importance of higher educational qualifications and the ability to work with other professional groups are nicely clarified by Gilliam Chumley (Chapter 3) who felt the best developments occurred when a multidisciplinary approach was adopted:

> In the last decade there has been a melding of nursing and medical roles within pain services. What was seen as the domain of the anaesthetist or physician has been cultivated and developed by nurses who are highly trained, often to a master or doctorate level, as I have been. Nurses have the advantage of working within the pain service full time and can devote more hours to its expansion. The role of the consultant nurse has allowed services to advance a stage further by treating their own clinical caseload and having designated time for education and research. That is not to say that nurses should work in isolation; the best developments occur when there is a multidisciplinary approach.

The ability to work effectively in an interprofessional team is fundamental but not without difficulties with different professional cultures inherent within the organisation (Hall 2005). Trudy Towell (Chapter 10) reflects on the study by Stenner and Courtenay (2008), who found that a lack of understanding of nurse prescribing among health care professionals could be a barrier:

> [T]his reflected my experiences where there was a lack of medical staff understanding of nurse prescribing and the knowledge base required. This can create a barrier as staff are not working seamlessly across boundaries as they do not understand each others roles and responsibilities.

The confidence to reach out to other professional groups and include them in the process of change was highlighted by Paul Bibby (Chapter 8) as he developed a new community service:

> Following an interim appraisal I approached GP practices and consulted directly about the service. It was clear from this that as the evidence suggests, GPs felt more involved and able to stake their claim in this project.

Similarly Ruth Day and Dee Burrows (Chapter 7) capture the importance of the ANP being able to work with patients, professionals and carers to form alliances which traditionally would have been undertaken by doctors:

> Claire demonstrates not just clinical expertise (which is expected from a clinical nurse specialist) but also an ability to bring people together (patient, healthcare professionals and carers) to form an alliance which supports the patient. This is a development clearly called for in the ANP competencies. It is one which some years ago might have been undertaken by doctors, but the development of

different roles in nursing has given us the opportunity to develop these alliances in a much more transparent fashion, using the latent leadership skills of senior clinical nurses.

A further important component of activity of those engaged in advancing practice was their involvement in interprofessional education. They often possessed a high level of knowledge and understanding of their subject and were keen to contribute to changing knowledge and attitudes. Eileen Mann (Chapter 4) identifies the importance of making this contribution:

> They may also be called upon to become more closely involved in the pain education of other health care professionals.

Interprofessional learning has been described as the process being where two or more professions purposely interact in order to learn with, from and about each, and this interaction can ultimately lead to improved effectiveness and the quality of care (Centre for the Advancement of Interprofessional Education 2002). This is, however, often difficult to attain in some circumstances because of professional differences. Referred to as tribalism (Beattie 1995), traditional educational and professional needs evolved separately with deep-rooted boundaries between them (Baxter & Brumfitt 2008), the result being a different practical and philosophical approach to patient care. Whilst training and learning often meant intraprofessional independence and autonomy, current policy changes in health care provision has meant that there is a blurring of roles and a role redesign to offer greater flexibility to meet patient demand (Skills for Health 2006; Baxter & Brumfitt 2008). A number of studies have evaluated the effectiveness of interprofessional education, some reaching the conclusion that in certain cases it proves to be beneficial. In a pilot study to assess the effectiveness of interprofessional pain workshops, Carr *et al.* (2003) found that interprofessional practitioner learning was positively evaluated and that knowledge transfer between the professional groups meant an increase in pain assessment and a reduction in pain referrals to the acute pain team. What this signifies that not only does interprofessional education and learning work but it also means a positive outcome for patients experiencing acute and chronic pain. This is clearly evident in Ann Taylor's work (Chapter 11) where she developed a masters programme in pain management. Comments from the nursing team demonstrated an overwhelming confidence in being able to deliver effective pain management and IPE was crucial to this development. Ann comments:

> . . . the nurses were able to construct knowledge based on what they had gained from the course and their own intuitions in order to make sense of themselves and their practice. All the nurses spoke of being more mature and having improved self-esteem and all described instances where they no longer had to rely on external validation for their self-identity. The nurses spoke of the knowledge they had constructed in providing them with an improved ability to care and described the continued use of frameworks to underpin practice. These frameworks were constructed by the nurses and were based upon their experiences and knowledge of interprofessional pain management, and they felt more satisfied in

their clinical roles. The nurses now perceived themselves as being part of a team rather than outside it; they felt valued, respected and capable. The nurses spoke of making connections that helped tie together pockets of knowledge and spoke of understanding that all knowledge was relative. The nurses wanted nursing to be seen as important in the care of patients in pain and spoke of making a difference; they now wanted to be respected for being nurses. Armed with the academic knowledge, confidence and self-worth, they provided examples of how they impacted on the care of patients in pain. (Ann Taylor)

There is an underlying theme within Ann's work that incorporates not only the educational perspective but also the interprofessional collaboration that ensures patient needs are effectively catered for. It is through this socialization of professional, cultural and attitudinal beliefs where the improvement in services stems from. In addition, Carr *et al.* (2003) suggested that key to delivering interprofessional pain education should ideally be the targeting of patients and their families to ensure acceptance of inadequate pain relief becomes a thing of the past.

Advancing practice in pain management

What we have attempted to portray in this book is that advancing practice encompasses many guises from the development of nurse-led clinics to entrepreneurial incentives that not only enhance patient care and outcome but development of the profession. The major themes to emerge have centred on clinical leadership, crossing the nursing–medical boundary and interprofessional team working. Providing an alternative approach to knowing-how and knowing-that allowed us to identify the knowledge required for advancing practice. We make the distinction that advancing practice involves a number of different facets and knowing-that is based on a choice of action which is informed from knowing-how, knowing-why and knowing-what (Chapter 1), a different perspective than those of Ryle (2000) and Rolfe (1998). What is crucial is the integration of the knowing-how knowledge into and supporting the knowing-that; the latter cannot function without a full appreciation and understanding of the former. It can be noticeable in some individual practitioners whereby they have neither developed nor can make those theoretical and practical links, for example a diabetic nurse may know everything to do with diabetes but fail notice when her patient becomes hypoglycaemic (the knowing-why), or a critical care nurse's ability to change a tracheostomy dressing (the knowing-how) and finally a surgical nurse observing cardiac arrhythmias but not able to identify the causative factors (the knowing-what). Therefore, in order for knowing-that to become meaningful, it is an amalgamation of these three facets and having done so can be judged to be advancing practice.

It has become evident that a dichotomy exists not only between what advancing and advanced practice are, but also within the concept of advanced practice itself. This can be explained by the very nature of what constitutes advancing and advanced practice. The rhetoric within the literature identifies who advanced practitioners are, either by role definition or by the attributes of the individual. Not readily explained is what actually constitutes advanced practice, nor is a practical definition offered of either advancing or advanced practice. This has invariably led to the confusion as to what advancing and advanced practices are. As a result, we have developed a working definition of advancing practice to challenge the current discourse and define it as:

> The ongoing procedural development of problem-solving, analytical and synthesis skills which allow practitioners to integrate practical knowing-how, theoretical knowing-why and experiential knowing-what into a pragmatic knowing-that knowledge to improve patient care/user need.

Important features within this definition are the three themes which are central to advancing practice: the practical/experiential and theoretical knowledge and the integration of this knowledge into a purposeful, autonomous knowing-that knowledge. There are some difficulties in defining practical/experiential knowledge because this is seen within the domain of practice and is often perceived as the hands-on, observational and social interaction knowledge that develops over time (Benner 1984; Rolfe *et al.* 2001; Estabrooks *et al.* 2005). This type of knowledge could be likened to what Carper (1978) refers to as aesthetic knowing or similar to Benner's (1984) intuitive knowing, knowledge which is gained through the 'gut feeling' type of experience and in which knowledge is a gathering process of scattered details and particulars of practice combined into an experienced whole, or equated with gaining knowledge through the use of experiential, practical patient cases (Benner 1984*)*. This experience provides a rich case study base of knowledge to be drawn upon. There are some notable similarities between these different perceptions of practical knowledge in that this could easily be compared with the work of the expert practitioner attributes which were mentioned previously. However, Fulbrook (2003) put forward the notion that knowledge to inform practice is contained within a variety of different sources, methods and methodologies. He referred to this as pragmatic epistemology which:

> . . . is about practical knowledge which incorporates all forms of knowing – it is the utilisation of knowledge within a practice setting: the value of knowledge for practice and the value of knowledge generated from practice. (Fulbrook 2003, p. 301)

Therefore, what Fulbrook (2003) is that clinical experience/expertise together with a diverse approach to 'evidence-based practice' culminates in effective patient care and improved practice. Whilst agreeing with Fulbrook (2003) in principle, the application of pragmatic knowledge in this context goes beyond his definition because what is important in terms of advancing practice is the *integration* of the different types of knowing and the understanding associated with this – the link between thinking and doing. Developing a mixture of knowing-how (practical knowing), knowing-why (theoretical knowing) and knowing-what (pattern recognition) leads to knowing-that – the choice of action determined by the practitioner's understanding of the situation.

Conclusions

Therefore, what is ever present throughout the book is that advancing practice in pain management is encapsulated in our concept of advancing practice as being a developmental process. It is easy to see that the knowing-how knowing-that framework can be used to define almost any aspect of nursing practice. Indeed, if one were to consider this framework outside of nursing per se, then its versatility is transferable to any profession. But it is within nursing that this framework has its founding. Unlike medicine, the pragmatic approach that many of the authors have illustrated here goes a long way in establishing nursing as a rising profession in health care provision. Some critics may argue that these are mere examples of nurses taking on the roles of medical colleagues. However, we suggest that it is the innovative and creative aspects of care provision that are being portrayed here. Admittedly, nursing is potentially at a cross-road with the opportunity to really grab opportunities for leadership. Too often time is wasted trying in discussion rather than getting on with the developments and as such we are attempting to highlight the importance of sharing experiences which not only demonstrate the competencies but also capture the complexity and reality of these initiatives through knowledge, skills and attitudes and therefore able to facilitate in unleashing the potential.

References

Baxter, S.K., Brumfitt, S.M., 2008. Professional differences in interprofessional working. *Journal of Interprofessional Care*, 22(3), 239–251.

Beattie, A., 1995. War & peace among health tribes. In Soothill, K., Mackay, L., Webb, C. (eds), *Interprofessional Relations in Health Care*, pp. 11–26. London: Edward Arnold.

Benner, P., 1984. *From Novice to Expert: Excellence and Power in Clinical Nursing Practice.* New York: Addison Wesley Publishing.

Cain, L.B., 2005. Essential qualities of an effective clinical leader. *Dimensions of Critical Care Nursing*, 24(1), 32–34.

Carper, B.A., 1978. Fundamental patterns of knowing. *Advances in Nursing Science*, 1(1), 13–23.

Carr, E.C.J., Brockbank, K., Barrett, R.F., 2003. Improving pain management through interprofessional education: evaluation of a pilot project. *Learning in Health and Social Care*, 2(1), 6–17.

Centre for the Advancement of Interprofessional Education, 2002. Defining interprofessional education. Available at http://www.caipe.org.uk/about-us/defining-ipe/?keywords=commission [accessed 11 May 2009].

Department of Health, 2000a. *A Service for All Talents: Developing the NHS Workforce.* Consultation Document on the Review of Workforce Planning. London: Department of Health.

Department of Health, 2000b. *NHS Plan: A Plan for Investment, a Plan for Reform.* London: Department of Health.

Department of Health, 2004. *The NHS Knowledge and Skills Framework (NHS KSF) and the Development Review Process.* London: Department of Health.

Department of Health, 2008. *A High Quality Workforce: NHS Next Stage Review.* London: Department of Health.

Estabrooks, C.A., Rutakumwa, W., O'Leary, K.A., Profetto-McGrath, J., Milner, M., Levers, M.J., Scott-Findlay, S., 2005. Sources of practice knowledge amongst nurses. *Qualitative Health Research*, 15(4), 460–476.

Fulbrook, P., 2003. *The Nature of Evidence to Inform Critical Care Nursing Practice*. Unpublished PhD thesis, Bournemouth University.

Hall, P., 2005. Interprofessional teamwork: professional cultures as barriers. *Journal of Interprofessional Care*, 19(S1), 188–196.

Por, J., 2008. A critical engagement with the concept of advancing nursing practice. *Journal of Nursing Management*, 16, 84–90.

Rolfe, G., 1998. Education for the advanced practitioner. In Rolfe, G., Fulbrook, P. (eds), *Advanced Nursing Practice*, pp. 271–280. Oxford: Butterworth-Heinemann.

Rolfe, G., Freshwater, D., Jasper, M., 2001. *Critical Reflection for Nursing and the Helping Professions: A Guide*. Basingstoke: Palgrave Macmillan.

Royal College of Nursing, 2003. *Nurse Practitioners: An RCN Guide to the Nurse Practitioner Role, Competencies and Programme Accreditation*. London: RCN.

Ryle, G., 2000. *The Concept of Mind*. London: Penguin Books.

Siriwardena, N., 2006. Releasing the potential of health services: translating clinical leadership into healthcare quality improvement. *Quality in Primary Care*, 14, 125–128.

Skills for Health, 2006. *Delivering a Flexible Workforce to Support Better Health and Health Services – The Case for Change*. Bristol: Skills for Health.

Stenner, K., Courtenay, M. 2008. The role of interprofessional relationships and support for nurse prescribing in acute and chronic pain. *Journal of Advanced Nursing*, 63(3), 276–283.

United Kingdom Central Council, 1994. *The Future of Nursing Practice. The Council's Standards for Education and Practice Following Registration: Position Statement on Policy and Implementation*. London: United Kingdom Central Council.

Index